WELL - WELL - WELL

EAT WELL

THINK WELL

LIVE WELL

FORWARD

Warm greetings, thank you for purchasing & taking the time to read this informative book. We are not expert professionals in any of the subjects we talk about. We have zero qualifications in nutrition, medication, or any other form of medical treatments.

Rather, we have over 138years of combined experience in all aspects of well being, stress free living. We do not take any type of medication, live in a joyful state of mind & continually seek the best ways to maintain & live a healthy, wealthy lifestyle.

Along our life's journey we have seen family, friends & acquaintances suffer & die too soon from lack of knowing the correct path to take when it came to their health & wellbeing. All put their faith in the medical establishment & although they are an essential part of our daily lives, most treat symptoms of illness, rather than seek cause & effect of any disease.

They say; God helps them who help themselves & with the information in this book, you can help yourself to put the percentage in your favor, to live out your life in true wellness & inspirational, joyous state of mind.

Before any lifestyle changes, you must first seek professional advice, for we live in a world that requires expert approval for any change can be sanctified. That said, the best cure is prevention & the more we learn what works & what doesn't, the better life we will live... Enjoy!

PART ONE

EAT WELL

Wisdom in Food, Nutrition in thought.

There is always a slew of advice on how to lose weight or how to eat a healthy diet. In most case, fad diets never work because they are hard to maintain. They just give a quick fix then within a few months or years, the dieter will return to the way they were eating before starting the diet. This is because the taste buds have a memory & high fat, sugar or salt foods that tend to lure a person back into old eating habits. Also, emotional eating when under stress is a major cause of overeating the wrong type of foods with high saturated fats, refined sugar and table salt.

Natural foods from nature contain the wisdom the mind and body need to stay healthy. Not all people are born physically equal...Some people are born with stronger genes & DNA so their bodies can tolerate more unhealthy foods and live to a ripe old age thanks in part to medical science. Therefore it makes sense to understand how you feel after eating each meal and to become aware of what your body can accept to stay healthy.

What thoughts do you have when you are ready for your next meal, doughnuts and coffee, full English breakfast, a tasty hamburger and French fries, or a juicy steak and jacket potato fully laden? Do you plan in advance your next meal whether it suits your taste buds or is going to make all the cells in your body rejoice?

When we look around, we see the majority of people hanker after a tasty meal, most probably high in fat, sugar and salt. Some people don't eat healthy but eat smaller portions to keep slim and then there are a few people that eat high nutrition, low calorie foods and stop eating just before they are full.

When junk food becomes a habit, over time most people will feel the effects that lead to diabetes, cancer and many other debilitating diseases. The pharmaceutical industry can dish out over-the-counter and prescription drugs that temporarily relieve painful digestive system discomfort but only a change of lifestyle will bring about a lasting cure.

Be aware, no matter how good a diet is, if a person thinks in a negative manner, especially when eating, the healthiest diet in the world can turn toxic. That said, it is far better to eat a healthy diet. A junk food diet only adds stress to the body and forms a chemical imbalance. A healthy diet rebalances the bodies digestive system & helps the immune system to function naturally

In the follow pages you will learn the authentic choices you have to stay healthy & joyful all your life. It is filled with tasty food choices and recipes containing natures wisdom you can enjoy, once you learn how to retrain your taste buds into accepting a truer way to eat. It usually takes 21 days to unhook from one unhealthy taste and change to a better choice.

Because most people have built-up multiple tastes, it takes time to change, so be patient and kind to yourself while making the changes slowly.

Emotional stress tends to lead to overeating foods with empty calories that contain little goodness, with a high calories count that adds weight rapidly... calories that have no benefit for the body but taste good while partaking in an overeating binge, trying to overcoming stressful situations.

It truth, it only makes matters far more stressful, for not only is a persons mind stressed by circumstances, the eating of junk food is also stressing out their bodies natural systems.
Respect what you put into mind & body & make a friend for life, abuse it with junk food-n-thoughts & become your own worst enemy.

Changing diets

A ' diet' is a way of eating, it can be a weight gain or loss diet, macrobiotic or vegan diet. When you decide it's time to get back in shape it's time to re-evaluate the foods one eats, which foods are health giving, which foods are empty calories, which foods have soluble fiber, which have non-soluble fiber (high fiber foods move slower through the body therefore giving a full feeling longer) All fruits and vegetables have fiber, soft drinks and fruit juices do not.

It usually takes years to gain and maintain excessive weight, so it is not possible to lose the weight in six months and keep it off. Have a realistic time plan, depending how much you weight you want to reduce.

To start the pathway to good health adapt the mind into thinking about the new foods you are going to be exploring and the old, unhealthy foods to start reducing. Often people eat when they are not hungry but feel the need to eat out of emotional stress. This type of hunger is called **emotional hunger** & is one of the main causes of obesity.

Reducing the high fat and high sugar foods with a health giving food, increasing the ratio gradually, eventually you will feel so much better, you will naturally stop eating the foods which are not health giving.

A golden rule about cooking, avoid frying any type of food. Steam or boil vegetables. Only use unsaturated oils such as virgin cold pressed olive oil in salad dressings.

Changing the desires of the taste buds takes 21 days for one type of food. If you decided to first reduce sugar intake, delete a food with high sugar, for example a donut, for 21 days. If after that time you desire a taste, have a bite or two, chew it very slowly. Small amounts will satisfy the desire, in time, you will not even want a taste, for when you increase the healthy foods the body desires, the healthier food leaves the body feeling satisfied, it also improves digestion and elimination.

To have good digestion your gut has to be healthy, it is necessary to take a probiotic pill daily, unless you eat a fresh, raw organic diet.

If you suffer any type of discomfort after eating it could mean any of the following

Eating on the run.

Foods you are unable to digest fully.

Eating whilst anxious.

Not chewing the food fully and overeating.

It is important to keep the body hydrated with fluids. This can come from fruit, vegetables and drinking at least 6 glasses of water a day. Be careful with fruit juices as they have a high sugar content with no fiber to slow the sugar down.

Having a glass of water 30 minutes before a meal will hydrate your body so you have no need to drink during your meal as this will reduce digestive acids. Room temperature water is easier on the body.

When having a meal take the time to sit at a table. Turn off TV, radio, computer that takes your attention away from the food you are eating. Turn on soft relaxing music that helps soothe your mind while your eating. Take time to smell your food before eating, this helps your digestive juices to start working.

The tip of the tongue is where the taste buds reside so the more time spent chewing the more flavor you acquire, digestive juices in the tongue start the first phase of digestion making it easier for the stomach to digest

Chew at least 30 times, if you have mindfulness when eating this will become one of your good habits when eating. This makes swallowing slower, therefore you can feel when you have eaten enough food. Eating quickly does not get the digestive juices working adequately, you swallow before the stomach has worked up enough digestive juices and this can lead to discomfort after you have finished eating.

It is preferable not to have any controversial conversation when eating as this can lead to a bloated stomach & gas.

Raw food provides enzymes which helps digestion, that is why it is good to start a meal with salad with minimum dressing, a little olive oil & balsamic vinegar helps the body to absorb the foods nutriments.

Overcooked food has less nutrition than less cooked or raw food. Raw food has the most nutrition except in a few cases e.g. tomatoes and carrots. If possible eat half raw food and half cooked Try to mix the colors of vegetables to get an assortment of vitamins and minerals

Elimination of food on a regular basis is an important function to clear toxic waste from the body. High fiber foods should be part of a daily diet. If constipation becomes a problem, take a natural laxative that contains organic ingredients but don't depend on it for too long.

Myths About Foods

You require dairy for your calcium needs.
Question: does a cow drink milk... No calves drink milk, the lucky cows eat grass. The unlucky ones are fed on corn & many injected with hormones & antibiotics. Many are kept in barns like battery hens. It's best to avoid all dairy products as they do effect the sinus & can cause cellulite in the body. Calcium is in most vegetables, especially green leafy, kale being one of the best sources.

All red meat products should be avoided as animal fats are a major cause of heart disease but if you must eat meat, only eat 100% grass fed.

Bananas are high in sugar.
If you compare them with an apple, yes. If you compare them with a piece of apple pie, no.

Avocados are high in fat.
The fat in an avocado is essential for bodily requirements. They are good nutrition for brain health.

Beans cause gas.
Soak beans all day, rinse and leave overnight, this starts the bean germinating and also takes less time to cook. Also boil the beans for five minutes, discard water and refill, cook until soft with fennel, ginger, turmeric, etc.

Vegetables cause gas
If your body is not used to eating raw vegetables, which is the most nutritious way to eat them, it may cause gas, start with a small quantity until gradually you body gets used to them and you shouldn't have a problem.

Truths About Food

Whole Grains ...the best grains are original and heirloom which have not been scientifically altered. Most wheat is refined and bleached into white flour. It is probably why there are so many allergies connected to glutton. If a person is allergic to glutton before changing their diet consult with a medical doctor who also uses alternative methods of treating patients. Try some of these grains and sense how better they make you feel ...

Grains

Amaranth...an ancient Aztec grain with superior nutrition. Rich in lysine and high quality protein. Gluten free. Goes rancid fast so store in fridge. Is available in black, red and white grains.

Whole barley... Superior to pearl as it retains it's bran, germ and endosperm. Higher in protein, calcium and potassium than pearl barley. (all barley is milled to some degree to remove 2 inedible husks}

Barley flakes....lightly toasted barley until soft and then pressed with steel rollers. Like rolled oats, barley flakes are great in cookies, breads, casseroles and for thickening soups

Buckwheat raw...gluten free high in 8 essential amino acids, high calcium, vitamin E and B vitamins. For a nutty flavor dry roast before boiling.

Bulgur wheat...let sit covered for 5-10 minutes after cooking. Bulgur is parboiled wheat berries, which is a star in the middle Eastern dish tabouli.

Couscous ...made from coarsely ground pre-cooked semolina. Couscous is a refined durum wheat.
Couscous whole wheat...fluff and let stand after cooking. More nutritious than the above.

Kamut...an ancient Egyptian wheat from 4000BC. It has a rich buttery, chewed texture. Up to 30% protein! rich in magnesium, zinc and vitamin E. Contains gluten but like many old original grains (not tampered with by humans) many wheat sensitive people eat it without reaction
Also made into flakes.

Millet...gluten free, alkaline which makes it easy to digest. Rich in lysine, a high quality protein and high in B vitamins. For a toasted taste, dry cook in saucepan until it pops, then add water.

Oat grouts...hulled with the bran and germ intact. All forms of oats are high in b vitamins, high quality protein . Oats have 4 times the fat as wheat, a natural antioxidant helps prevent rancidity. The high fat content makes it creamy. Good for breakfast, pilafs and dough

Rolled oats...oat grouts crushed between steel rollers, quicker to cook, Soaked for several hours or overnight reduces cooking time considerably.

Quinoa.. Pronounced keen-wah Must be rinsed thoroughly in a sieve under running water to remove a bitter taste which protects the seed from birds .
A very high quality grain, high protein, more iron, phosphorus, vitamins A E and B and more calcium and fat than other grains.

Rye berries....higher in protein, phosphorus, iron and potassium than wheat. High in lysine, low in gluten, high in fiber and has special long chains of sugars which digest slowly and provide long lasting energy. Also in flakes.

Spelt berries... a light fluffy and nutty flavor called faro in Italy an un hybridized bread wheat, eaten around the world for over 5000 years.

Teff berries, a cross between rye and wheat

Brown/wild rice

Before cooking grains, rinse thoroughly in cold water until water runs clear.

Strain them to remove any dirt or debris. Cooking times on packet.

Presoaking can reduce cooking time by 40%.

Bring to boil, add grain and return to boil.

Reduce and simmer.

Lifting lid whilst cooking loses steam.

Most grains are slightly chewy when cooked

Beans

Modern day illnesses have come about by highly processed foods, high in salt, sugars and fats which are low in nutrients, thus requiring a greater intake of empty calories to maintain the needs of the body to keep functioning.

Beans and grains have been used in cooking for thousands of years, they are high in fiber, high in nutrients and low in fat. They are recommend by the America Heart Association for a heart healthy diet. They can be stored for many years and are only activated when coming into contact with water.

Beans contain a high protein content, low in fat and high in fiber, high in nutrients. Even though some beans are higher in fat than others, all beans have far less fat than animal products and vegetable fats and the sugars enter the blood stream much slower due to the high fiber content, thus keeping you satisfied longer. These are a good alternative to meat or chicken, if paired with grains to make 9 amino acids.

Some beans are harder to digest than others.
Even if a bean or grain says no soaking necessary, soaking for a few hours lowers the cooking time and washers away any inhibitors the bean or grain may have (an inhibitor is on the bean or grain to stop the birds eating the seeds and prevents it from sprouting until it comes in contact with water).

For beans that require soaking over night, after soaking boil for five minutes then discard the water. Use fresh water and continue cooking, add some sliced ginger at this time. Twenty minutes before the end of cooking add onions, carrots and celery to add flavor. Also at this time add toasted spices or a curry powder. Salt is best added at the end of cooking if you require it. Over time you will find the spices add a nice flavor (coriander , cumin, cardamom fennel, anise etc.)
If you like a touch of heat add chili peppers .

Aduki bean...no soaking necessary. These are easier to digest than many beans, low in fat. Good for the kidneys.

Anasazi bean...a revived heirloom bean related to the pinto bean but much sweeter holds it's shape during cooking, low in fat.

Black-eyed peas. Quick cooking, after being soaked and a good source of selenium. Easily digested.

Black beans, very popular. High in magnesium, low in fat

Dal...dahl....like a split pea only smaller. Used in Indian cooking...no need to soak.

Camellia beans or white kidney beans..

Fava or broad beans ...peel off skins after soaking.

Garbanzo beans or chickpeas...very flavorful whole or made into hummus...great for sprouting.

Great northern beans...

Kidney beans...holds it shape well.

Lentils...red, green and brown. No soaking necessary red lentils cook quickly and lose shape...green lentils are great for sprouting

Mung beans...soaking not necessary. Used in Indian cuisine...easy to digest, thickens when cold...great sprouting.

Navy beans..soaking necessary. Used for making baked beans.

Peas whole, soaking necessary. ..can be used in soup and dips or as mushy peas.

Peas split...no soaking necessary, creamy texture, good as dips or soup.

Pinto beans...used for re- fried beans.

Red beans...smaller than kidney bean.

Soy beans...sweet nutty flavor, exceptional health benefits. Add salt to water to keep skins on. The only legume containing 9 essential amino acids, a complete protein, and a higher fat content.

Alternative ideas for using beans, mix and match.
Add cubed squash and Tamari for last half hour.

Toss beans with chopped onion, minced garlic and herbs.

Add tomato, onion, garlic and herbs of your choice.

Mash beans, add herbs of your choice, shape into patties, spray with a little olive oil and broil, or make into pate for serving on crackers or sandwiches.

Chopped onion, grated ginger and turmeric, cumin, coriander and cayenne. Let sit a few minutes before serving

Add black strap molasses for a different flavor, and provides calcium and iron

Toasted sesame seeds, chopped garlic, scallions, lemon juice, mint. Mash with ginger powder and cooked sweet potato.

Even when no soaking is required soak for up to 2 hours and rinse thoroughly, this also reduces cooking time.

High Antioxidant Foods

Antioxidants are natural substances that may stop or limit the damage caused by free radicals that are derived from exposure to too much oxygen that forms into harmful oxidation. Body chemicals alter to become free radicals. Pollution, tobacco smoke, alcohol, etc and too much sun exposure, create free radicals.

Over many years, free radicals can cause chain reactions in our body, damaging or destroying essential body chemicals, DNA and parts of our cell structure. Free radicals can contribute to faster aging, also they contribute to the onset of diseases such as; heart disease, cancer and diabetes to name a few of the many

Your body uses antioxidants to stabilize the free radicals. This keeps them from causing damage to other cells. Antioxidants can protect and reverse the damage caused by oxidation to some extent.
Some of the highest antioxidant foods are....

Red beans
Wild blueberries
Red kidney beans
Blueberries
Prunes
Raspberries
Strawberries
Apples
Sweet dark cherries
Pecans
Walnuts
Hazelnuts
Cloves
Cinnamon
Turmeric
Oregano

Top Healthy Foods to mix & match

Acai berry rich in glutathione -,steam lightly before eating

Almonds rich in calcium

Apples

Apple cider vinaigrette - un-pasteurized

Avocado

All dried beans. Some are easier to digest than others, soak during the day, rinse and allow to sprout overnight, this process makes them less gassy

Beet high in iron

Blueberries

Bilberries. (huckleberries)

Bitter melon, available in Chinese store helps recovery from type 2 diabetes

Broccoli

Cabbage & sauerkraut, red & green mixed together with added caraway seeds.

Carrots

Celery

Cherry

Dark Chocolate

Coconut

Cucumber

DHA and EPA food oil from fish, especially good sardines, mackerel, tuna and salmon.

Flax seeds, hemp seeds and chia seeds (a vegan alternative) all have good quality oils 3 and 9. most foods contain too much no 6

Eggs...in moderation

Egg plant.

Fresh green beans. high in L-dopa, eat 1-2 oz per day

Garlic

Ginger

White and green tea

Goji berry

Grapefruit, peel leaving as much pith as possible on the fruit, put in Vitamix with 3 frozen strawberries blend till creamy. 30-60 seconds. Cleansing.

Horsetail herb...good for bones

Kiwi

Limes

Maca powder, there are 3 types, white for increasing stamina, red to keep the prostate healthy and black, similar properties to white.

All types of mushrooms

Manuka honey has antibacterial activity ...bees collect the pollen from manuka, trees in New Zealand

Royal jelly and bee pollen, helps renew vitality

Propolis ... Synergistic honey blend, relief from sore throats and colds.

Natty powder...a fermented soy product helps in building bone.

Okra...the seeds contain mucilage which makes it a very good soluble fiber.

Olive oil

Papaya

Pineapple

Pears

Sesame oil raw and unrefined.

Spices, cinnamon, cardamom, cumin, turmeric, red peppers.

Swiss chard...eat raw in salads or smoothies.

Oranges

Onions...all types, the purple one being the most nutritious.

Papaya...good for digestion.

Pineapple ...good for digestion

Pomegranate...heart healing

Pumpkin seed ...rich in zinc, good for prostate

Raspberries

Raw chocolate beans, for happy and healthy vibes

All sea vegetables...broader range of minerals than other food

Sesame seeds

Spinach

Squash family

Organic strawberries

Purple and red potatoes

Kale, no 1 of all greens, use raw in salads or lightly steamed.

Watercress aids in the absorption of iron.

Tomato

Turmeric

Walnut...king of nuts

Watermelon...a great cleansing fruit

Wheat germ high form of vitamin E

Rosemary...kept normal cells from mutating in rats.

Cilantro helps cleanse heavy metals.

Turmeric to control inflammation.
Spirulina, a highly nutritious seaweed

When eating an organic, high nutrition diet supplements should not be required.

Foods & Drink To Delete From Your Shopping List

Alcohol - all alcoholic drinks are high in sugar & can adversely effect every cell in the body & brain as alcohol is a registered poison. Avoid at all costs

Sugar - Large intake of sugar over time causes cancer & many other debilitating diseases. Avoid added white sugar in all foods & keep well away from all sugar substitutes.[many of which can be harmful over a period pf time] The sugar in whole foods is digested at a slower pace in the body due to the fiber content, juices are not a healthy alternative to water,

White bread; white processed flour, white processed sugar and white processed salt. All have all the minerals and fiber removed thus making them void of the nutrients that a healthy body requires.
Most mass produced breads contains bromide to extend shelf life & other unhealthy ingredients. A better alternative is Ezekiel bread found in freezer dept of most supermarkets. It is made of sprouted grains.

Hydrogenated oils - manufacturers are now removing this type of fat from their foods as it has been proven that it is detrimental to good health. Check all labels to make sure.

High fructose corn syrup - is proven to be detrimental to health.

Canola oil - a GMO product which is detrimental to good health. It has been linked to heart attacks and cancer.
Alternative...organic coconut oil or olive oil

Cold cuts - which are highly salted and contain nitrates. If eating any type of meat only eat fresh cooked, organic fed.

Meat that is not organic could possibly contain estrogen, antibiotics and pesticides. Compound reared cows are fed corn, kept in overcrowded pens and require antibiotics to keep them free of disease. Cows grazed in open fields, the old fashioned way (unfortunately not all grass fed are equal...many are taken to the compound for the last 3-6 months and fed corn to fatten them up). When buying meat only eat 100% grass fed and eat smaller portions

Chicken - keep clear of battery hens, look for free range organic fed hens if you must eat meat.

Dairy products - cause mucus in the sinuses & cellulite on the legs & butt. Aged cheeses may cause headaches in some people & can causes blocked arteries and calcium deposits .in the wrong places. Cheese is very constipating along with white store bought bread. The countries with the most osteoporosis consume the highest amount of milk and cheese.
you may find many benefits not having dairy & fewer allergies

Canned goods -Many are usually high in salt & sugar, so read the label. If you can't find fresh food then choose your product carefully & only eat organic tinned foods

Soda - all sodas are like drinking poison water, they also deplete calcium from the bones.

.**Food preservative** - are very beneficial for the supermarkets as the food can be on the shelves for quite a while with no spoilage . They may be good for the bottom line but not for a healthy system. Fresh foods have a very short shelf life, therefore cost more, but your body will appreciate having 'clean' food.
Many tests have bean done on nitrates in almost all cooked meats & they are not recommended.

Red meat - clogs the arteries leading to heart disease

7 Foods that can cause allergies

Peanuts...soy...sugar...corn...eggs...dairy...gluten

Foods to eat regularly

As many leafy greens as you desire

A selection of any vegetables

Moderate amounts of fresh fruit (all fruit contains sugar, the fiber slows the digestion therefore does not spike insulin as much as added sugar)

All grains (soak overnight and then cut down on cooking time)

All beans and legumes (soak both overnight, rinse in the morning and rinse again before using, if you are cooking later in the day)

All organic seeds & nuts produce probiotics when soaked in pure water, rinsed & left to dry, unless they have been irradiated.

Home made bread made of wholesome sprouted nuts and seeds is the best solution. In the morning place the amount of seeds you require in glass jars and cover with water, In the evening drain and rinse, leave to sprout overnight, fill the jar with water, shake well and drain. Place seeds on baking tray and leave to dry. When fully dry place in freezer. When frozen grind the seeds in a Vitamix blender or a grinder. Soaking the seeds removes the inhibitors that are in all seeds that prevents them from sprouting until they are watered. This also changes the seed into a living food with a hundred times more nutrients. Lightly toasting bread makes it more digestible....see recipe for yeast less bread in a later chapter .

Foods to Ward Off Disease

Two of the most powerful healing foods are wheat grass and Rejuvelac

Winter Wheat is a grain that when sprouted produces wheatgrass.

Wheatgrass juice is liquid chlorophyll full of vitamins and minerals. Combining wheatgrass with a healthy diet will restore lost health

Wheat grass contains A, B-complex, C, E, and K and minerals calcium, iron, magnesium, phosphorus, sulphur, and zinc. It contains all 17 essential amino acids. Enzymes and amino acids are responsible for cell renewal.

Drink wheatgrass on an empty stomach and wait 20 minutes before eating.

There should be no problem with wheat allergies as only the plant is being used. Wheatgrass is easy to digest and a great nourishing "medicine' for the body.

Wheat grass creates an unfavorable environment for bacteria to grow, making it an effective healer.

There are many reports from scientists showing all the nutrients necessary for normal body function could be found in many weeds and grasses. The lucky cows survive on grass and hay

When you start to eat more plant foods your body starts to detoxify, which in some cases can cause headaches, diarrhea, mucous, etc. if you slowly add more plant food and cut down on meats and dairy products the affects will not be so drastic. If your body has been compromised with bad health cutting out all harmful foods may be necessary and cleansing drinks made from organic foods like kale, celery, cucumber, spinach and wheatgrass shots, making sure you have regular bowel movements so the waste is leaving your body. A qualified health care person should be consulted.

Wheat grass can be bought from a whole food market and you juice it at home and drink immediately. One portion is about two fluid ounces.

If you do not have a juicer put a handful of wheat grass in the blender, strain and drink. The grass should taste sweet.

Wheatgrass can be grown in the house or on the patio. The cooler months are the best time for growing.

Soak a cupful of seeds in a large jar overnight

Next day rinse and drain and place equal amounts in 3 jars

Rinse and drain twice a day for 2-3 days.

Place an unbleached paper towel in a large shallow ceramic or Pyrex dish sprinkling underneath the towel a teaspoon of powdered kelp (this is like fertilizer for the plant). Dampen the paper towel.

Spread the seedlings out in the dish.

Cover with a damp cloth (keep the cloth damp at all times) for 3 days until 2-3 inches tall. Check daily and if required spray with filtered waster.

Remove cloth and place in a light place and grow for 7-10 days, watering as required. Use filtered water.

As the dish does not have drainage do not let the plants stand in water.

Sometimes a fungus grows at the root, this is ok. When cutting for use cut above the fungus.

You can set the seeds every four days so you have a constant supply.

We do not use plastic or metal containers for growing or sprouting and always use filtered or good bottled water. Unfortunately most bottles used these days are plastic for most juices and water.

Cut as required and best used immediately.

Rejuvelac is a probiotic drink made from soft wheat berries or rye.

This can be an acquired taste as it is a little pungent with a sweaty sock taste. The quality of the seed and the temperature of the room can affect the taste, (If the room is over warm it is stronger). It is highly nutritious and healing, some times I add a squeeze of lemon and drink between meals or it can be used instead of water in a smoothie.

To make...place one cup of soft wheat berries or rye in a glass jar and fill with filtered water. Rinse the berries twice a day for one and a half -two days. This is important to avoid mold. When the tails of the seed are the same length as the seed rinse the berries 2 times, fill with water and soak for 48 hours. After 48 hours pour this into a container and drink or store in the refrigerator. Refill the seed jar with water, leave 24 hours and strain off, you can possibly do this 1 or 2 more times. The grains can then be fed to the birds. Do not compost them as they have been fermented.

Good rejuvelac is a cloudy, faintly yellow liquid with a tart, lemon like taste, is slightly carbonated with small bubbles. The tail on the sprout is important, if it is under sprouted it will taste weak and bitter. If the tail is too long it could be bitter or sweet. It's natural for a layer of foam to appear on top. This is not harmful

Manuka honey, which is from the Manuka tree has proven to kill the H.pylori bacteria along with healing cabbage juice, which is high in the amino acid glutamine. Keep using the cabbage juice until there is no pain from the ulcer. At this time eat only a vegan diet. No dairy or animal protein. If the pain continues see a health care practitioner/MD. Who can use holistic healing.

Vision Improvement

A diet lacking in the right nutrients is the cause of most modern day ailments, the eye is no different. In Chinese medicine the eyes are connected to the liver. We require good digestion and elimination to be able to absorb the nutrition from the food we eat and to eliminate all the waste products. The eyes require two carotenoids called zeaxanthin and lutein, which are phytochemicals The foods which contain the necessary nutrients are avocado, orange bell peppers, yellow corn, egg yolk, kale, carrots, tomatoes. Bilberries (also called huckleberries) are a great antioxidant available in capsules or whole dried powder.

High Blood Pressure

Add Garlic & Ginger to most meals as they are anti inflammatory, anti viral & help lower cholesterol & blood pressure.

Eat six stalks of celery each day it contains pthalides which help to relax the muscles around arteries and allow these blood vessels to dilate. Also follow a vegan diet. Celery has large amounts of pesticides so organic would be more favorable.

Reduce your salt intake by eliminating convenience foods with high salt & seldom add extra salt to your meals. If you need to add a little use Himalayan salt

Walnuts are full of good nutrients which help blood flow. They can be added to meals or eaten on their own. Soak for 2-3 hour before eating to remove the inhibitors which stop them sprouting.

Okra has special fibers and gums that pull fat out of the arteries. Eat a little each day added to a meal
Eggplant also has properties for cleansing the arteries.

Fatty fish such as salmon, mackerel , trout or sardine should be the protein of the day. They act as a blood thinner.
Pomegranate juice or fresh pomegranate are rich in antioxidants.

Fresh or fermented beets. Grate beets, onions and garlic, mix in a few caraway seeds, fill a glass jar, push down on beets and fill with unpasteurized cider vinegar. Put a table spoonful once a day on salads & vegetables.
The flesh of one avocado has more soluble fiber than a bowl of oatmeal. The fat is more beneficial than olive or almond oil. The seed can also be used in a smoothie.
Goji berries, maca powder and acai berries can be added to a smoothie.
Cut down on caffeinated drinks
green or white tea, mint tea, chamomile, oat straw and corn silk instead of coffee

Keeping Bones Strong

Calcium

The blood ph is always 7.4 if this is not maintained we would be dead. When a meal of protein is not balanced out with alkaline foods there is not enough calcium to neutralize the acid, so calcium is taken from the bones. If this is happening on a regular basis eventually the bones will be losing more calcium than is being replaced.

Plant calcium is more absorbable in all the right places, as nature intended. Watercress, Swiss chard, kale are high in calcium and magnesium. Also broccoli, cauliflower, Brussels sprouts , all cabbage etc. Cucumber is alkaline and silica rich, include this every day in the smoothies and in salads.

The herb horsetail provides silica, a mineral for increasing bone density, and also strengthening hair and nails. Horsetail can deplete the vitamin b-l. If you eat beans and grains on a regular basis this will be no problem

Interval walking/jogging is bone building, have a 30 second interval jogging when walking. When sitting for long periods, stand up if possible and bounce and shake for 2 minutes each hour. Bounce and shake...stand the feet shoulder width apart, knees slightly bent and gently bounce,

Hold arms in front with elbows bent and hands loose and shake. Do this for 2 minutes. Breathing deeply. This stimulates the lymph glands to cleanse and pumps the blood quicker around the body making you feel more alive and helps concentration.

Sunshine is necessary for the body in small doses, not laying out and baking. 20 - 30 minutes (preferably not between 11 am and 3

pm when it is at its strongest. Depending on where you live, of course).

If you are unwell then some sunshine will definitely improve your health. Cholesterol gets converted into vitamin D from sunlight.

People living in areas where there are low levels of sunlight have a greater level of osteoporosis and depression...sunlight enhances health.

Have short periods in the sunlight early morning or late afternoon without sun lotion. If this is not possible take a vitamin d3 capsules.

Cancers are caused by stress over time, diet over time and chemicals...do not fear a little sunshine daily, if possible. Allow short periods when the sun is not too-high to go without sunglasses.

Bearing in mind many sun lotions are cocktails of chemicals, a long sleeve shirt is better protection over long periods in the sun.

Getting a good tan looks good for a short time, then it fades and in the long term speeds up the aging of the skin.

The English rose ladies would wear long clothes, long sleeves, cotton gloves and large brimmed hats when they were stationed abroad with their army husbands in hot climates to keep their skin from aging from the sun.

We do require sunshine for good health, so use your own good judgment when enough is enough.

Gout & Arthritis

1 tablespoon of sour cherry concentrate and 1 teaspoon of Apple cider vinaigrette mixed in a full glass of water, will benefit the body for gout, arthritis and lack of energy.

Also the "magic" mix of chia, hemp, flax and buckwheat seeds, soaked overnight along with soaked walnuts.

This helps lubricate the joints with inflammation fighting prostaglandins.

Use 1/2 teaspoon of turmeric, as a seasoning on all your meals. Ginger and turmeric made into a tea occasionally adding licorice makes a soothing drink.

Licorice, should only be use for 2-3 times a week.

Asthma, Autism, Alzheimer's, Chronic Fatigue and Fibromyalgia, are correlated with high Mercury levels. The air we breath can be contaminated with Mercury and many other pollutants.

A dairy/gluten free diet with a high photochemical diet, made into tasty smoothies has been known to help them cope better with every day tasks.

AHCC. Is perhaps the worlds most researched immune supplement with 100 supporting research studies, showing the awesome cancer fighting properties in the elderly. It also used in hospitals in Japan that helps the immune system s response against MSRA

Germs/ Viruses are everywhere....the pen at the cashiers when signing credit cards, door handles, counter tops, library books & DVD's, handshakes, to name but a few places they lurk. Be aware of their existence wherever you may be. Never touch your face, eyes, nose, ears when out. Keep alcohol wipes in your bag or in the car & use them before starting home.

Dental Hygiene

It is said we dig our grave with our teeth, so why not change the dynamics of that statement and preserve our health with our teeth. To do that we need to have good dental hygiene. After every meal floss and brush your teeth and gums. The gums are just as important as the teeth, maybe more so, to keep in good condition. Brushing the gums stimulates them and keeps them healthy. Use a soft toothbrush. A little care can save a whole lot of trouble in the future.

Sleep considered by many people as an inconvenience but is essential for renewal & energy to take on the progress of the next days events whatever they may be.

To gain the full benefit of sleep an ideal bedtime is between 10 - 11 pm most nights. There are 4 grades of sleep know as sleep ram, the deeper the sleep the higher the ram grade.

Cellular repair time occurs generally between 10 pm and 2 am when a person with a relaxed, empty state of mind enjoys 4 ram of sleep which is considered to be the deepest for of sleep, with the best health befits.

Children are more likely to be in a deep state of sleep as their brains have not been developed long enough to absorb too many negative thoughts that keeps older folks awake, or in a in lower ram of sleep.

If you are going through an illness or feel groggy and tired most of the time and require caffeine to keep you going, cut it down and stop any caffeine drinks 5 hours before bedtime. Turn of the TV or radio two hour before bedtime & do not listen to any negative news during the day. Just catch up with the headlines and leave the negative news to those who are habitually hooked on it for a fix. You should try to get to bed by 10 pm.

6 - 8 hours sleep are required for a healthy person.

Too much sleep is not healthy, so everything in moderation.

On awakening have a glass of water to replenish the fluids you lost during the night.

Hot tea can also be taken with a little good quality raw honey. Processed honey is not the choice to make.

Breathing ... something we all do every minute or so but are we getting the most out of every breath?

Shallow breathing can make us feel sluggish. Become aware of how regular we deep breath.

Start by breathing in to the count of 6 hold for the count of 4 and blow out for the count of 8 Keep checking in on your breathing every few hours. Awareness of our breathing is an important factor in keeping the blood flowing though our body and the brain alert.

Relax The Brain Cells With Joyful Thoughts.

Live in love and joy... do not harbor feelings of hate and resentment. "Forgive those that have trespassed against us" are wise words from the bible.

Your health will benefit greatly by letting go of this baggage.

Holding on to feelings of grief, sadness, anger, resentment, frustration, guilt and fear...can destroy the love and joy of your wellbeing.

The hormones cortisol & adrenaline, when in excessive mode in our body can lead to destruction of the good cells & allow the onslaught of disease.

Stay away from scary things like horror movies, negative TV news channels and any situations that stimulates anger.

Keep oneself on a balance to keep good health....excess adrenal stimulation harms health.

Water

Get a good filtration system in your home & make sure you change the filters on a regular basis.

The body is 80% water... 6 - 8 glasses of water a day is recommended, if you are eating fruit and vegetables this is counted in with your quota. Drink green or white tea which has way less caffeine than black tea, fruit and herb teas and if you must drink coffee limit it to 1 or 2 cups a day. Alcohol is a registered poison and a diuretic that takes water from your body

If you suffer badly from arthritis using distilled water for 4 weeks may take some of the mineral deposits away from your sore joints. Adding a little sea salt or Himalayan salt will add absorbable minerals

Dried fruits ... drink more water if you are eating dried fruit
Nettle leaf tea first thing in the morning is helpful in lowering histamine levels.

Tips on Natural Choices For Better Health

As a reminder ...
All symptoms of illness require first class medical attention. None of the suggestions in this book are meant to take the place of doctors. The following choices are to prevent/relieve symptoms of illness & disease.

Arthritic joints...Turmeric is good at stopping nitric oxide which attacks the joints

Strengthen chest and lungs...sage and or thyme tea...2/3 cups daily
Aids digestion and sleep...mint tea

Low libido...add ginger...cloves...peppermint...Cinnamon ...star anise in teas and baths

High cholesterol ...oats...barley with husk, black or brown...garlic...Ginger...cayenne...celery

Insomnia...last meal of the day...oats...chamomile,

Sore eyes...cool cucumber...also good to eat

Heart attack... Call emergency services, then add lavender oil in fold of elbow and put an aspirin under tongue. Keep calm till help arrives.
Burns...lavender...then ice

Energy boosting, basil, rosemary, lemongrass, lemon, bergamot, grapefruit, aromatherapy oil.

Liver cleanse, milk thistle, yellow dock, dandelion, hormone rich garden sage. Walking relieves flatulence

Depression cut out caffeine and sugar as quickly as possible, St. Johns wart, magnesium rich foods, B vitamin supplement...lecithin. Where possible eat the appropriate foods. Calcium and silica (available from horsetail) in the diet prevents the absorption of aluminum to the brain
Cilantro...helps to clear heavy metals from the body

Prostate ... pumpkin seeds, saw palmetto, flaxseed, lycopene, bilberries, vitamin e, zinc

Chronic intestinal disorders...usually a lack of essential fatty acids. Try hemp seed, chia seeds, flax seeds, buckwheat seeds, either ground and sprinkled on food, or sprouted and used in a smoothie.

Colds with stuffy nose
Aromatherapy oils are very strong, one drop is adequate. Steam inhaler with one drop of oil, Olbas, peppermint or eucalyptus. Pour boiling water in a bowl, add 1 drop of any one of the above, cover head with towel and inhale, also alternate nostrils if one is more blocked than the other. Place the bowl on a firm surface and be careful not to tip the water over

Extra probiotics

Propolis capsules or propolis honey

Hot pepper flakes added to hot water

Make a drink of lemons, ginger and licorice and sip throughout the day.

Eat only cleansing foods. with garlic & ginger

Organic chicken soup made with extra onions, celery, carrots and garlic & ginger.

Deep breathing exercises throughout the day.

Take 1/2 teaspoon vitamin c powder in a glass of warm water and a zinc tablet 3-4 times a day.

Elderberry capsules and zinc tablets help to shorten a cold.
Add bacteria killing herb thyme to honey to make a cough syrup.

Blend 1 onion with 5-10 cloves garlic and Manuka honey. Take 2 teaspoons as is or in warm water?

For a sore throat gargle with salt and warm water at 1 hour intervals.

Make a concoction of sage and liquorices for a gargle

After 2-3 days the symptoms should be gone.

A runny nose is one way the body detoxes itself, especially if you have been eating high animal fat foods. Vegetarian fats are absorbed into the body and are health giving.

Some cough medicines can lower blood pressure. Follow the instructions carefully.

If the pain of the sore throat is unbearable suck on a pain relieving lozenge.

Headache

Morning headaches can be caused through jaw clenching or teeth grinding, which is caused by stress whilst you are sleeping. Do not take your worries and anxieties to bed with you. Before going to sleep relax your mind and body.

An exercise for relieving stress

Stress reducing exercise before going to bed
Relax the body by tensing the muscles in the upper arms, hold for 5 seconds, then release, tense the lower arm for 5 seconds and release, tense the fingers for 5 seconds and release, the same for the legs, buttocks, stomach, shoulders, neck and face, breathing in when tensing and blowing out on the release.

When this is complete slowly recite the poem; The Blissful Silence, or one of the other meditative poems found in the back pages of the book. Starting with the first verse and adding the rest when you have memorized it. You will find you fall into a deep blissful sleep and wake up really refreshed.

If you do have a headache, before reaching for the pill bottle use an ice pack or a bag of frozen peas, place the cold bag on the pressure points of the face, each side of the nose, lips, chin, front and back neck hold the bag on each point for 5 seconds before moving on to the next. At the same time, put a couple of drops of peppermint oil between the palms of your hands, rub them together and inhale, one nostril at a time.

For a sinus headache pour a small amount of boiling water into a bowl, put one drop of eucalyptus or Olbas oil in the water, place a towel over your head to hold in the steam and inhale several times, this helps to unblock the mucus in the sinus thus relieving the pressure. Use caution with using boiling water, place on a sturdy table away from the edge and sit on a chair.

For a tension headache, a drop of each of the following essential oils mixed with a small amount of carrier oil... Blue chamomile, frankincense, clary sage and lavender. (If you only have lavender use that) This will produce a calming effect for relaxation.

Migraine Headaches

Most common causes of headaches are ordinary foods people eat every day. Certain foods seem to be able to cause migraines, cluster headaches and tension headaches. The foods most likely to cause a headache are any food or drink with caffeine, aged cheese, alcohol (especially red wine) chocolate, aged or cured cold cut meats, gravy mix, soup mixes with hydrolyzed protein, MSG, yeast, sauerkraut, Kim chi and other aged foods, dried fruits, imitation crab, licorice, salty foods, rhubarb, yogurt, milk, wheat, many processed sauces. Read the ingredients of all prepared foods.

Remove all these foods from your diet for 60 days. After this time replace one food every two weeks. If after two weeks that food is okay, move onto the next food, sometimes the foods we crave the most are the culprit. Eating the same foods daily could build up to an intolerance. Vary the diet.

Apple Cider Vinegar [ACV] ... organic unpasteurized has friendly micro organisms to inhibit the growth of unfriendly organisms

ACV is excellent in dressings, for pickling and many home remedies.

For any yeast or fungal infection on the scalp or the soles of the feet, an ACV rinse seldom fails as a cure.

ACV is an old remedy that helps restore the body's pH to a healthy, mildly acidic state. When applying vinaigrette to the skin dilute it with equal amounts of water.

Apples are a rich source of potassium and pectin which helps to cleanse the intestines by absorbing toxins and enabling them to pass through the bowels.

Fights bacteria and viruses...1 teaspoon raw honey, 1teaspoon ACV in warm water...sip slowly

Purification...blend lightly cooked carrots and greens with ACV, eat between meals.

To release a headache...2 tablespoons ACV in boiling water...inhale vapors.
 Also put hot pepper flakes in hot water and sip. 1/4 - 1/2 teaspoon of peppers. ACV cold compress on back of neck.

Sore throats...1 teaspoon ACV in glass of warm water...gargle and spit out 3 times every hour. as throat feels easier gargle at 3 hourly intervals.

Compress on throat or lungs...place a thin cloth soaked in ACV place over throat and cover with Saran Wrap . Use hot towels on lungs

Skin...1/2 cup ACV in small basin of warm water...rub mixture all over skin till dry. Repeat twice a week.

Use only pure soaps on skin.

ACV is good on sunburn

Aloe gel is a good skin toner, excellent for sun burn.

Cleansing face...wash face with warm water, hold a hit cloth on face for 3 minutes. Soak thin cloth in 2 tablespoons ACV diluted in 1 cup water.

Place on face, cover with hot cloth. Lie with feet elevated for 10 minutes. Remove cloths, gently rub skin upwards with coarse cloth. Use once per week.

Apply to herpes sores.

Poison ivy, mosquito bites, beestings, jelly fish, swimmers ear...50/50 ACV and water.
Yeast infection

Dandruff...3 tablespoon in 1 cup water. Sponge onto scalp and leave for 30-120 minutes,

Wash and rinse in a diluted solution of ACV and water...leaves hair silky soft.

Use ACV as a hair conditioner, for dry, over bleached and broken hair Mix 2 - 4 tablespoons coconut oil, 1 tablespoon avocado oil, 3 - 4 tablespoons ACV. Mix together. Rub into scalp, leave on for 20 minutes or longer.

Wash out using non sulfated shampoo and conditioner. Use once a month.

ACV has the correct ph balance for the body. This works miracles.

Muscle soreness - aching joints... Relax in a tub, add 1cup ACV, massage entire body. Finish with finger tip massage of scalp

Improve digestion... 5 minutes before mealtime take 1/3 teaspoon ACV with 1 tablespoon water, hold in mouth a few minutes before swallowing. Also chew on fennel seeds...drink cabbage juice. Or make teas from... anise, cardamom, peppermint

Good for prostate...2 tablespoons ACV , 2 tablespoons olive oil a dash of amino acids, ground pumpkin seeds, use over salads and vegetables.

Mucus...remove dairy, eggs and sugar from diet,
 3 cocktails daily, ACV throat gargle, inhale ACV in boiling water and a fresh carrot and green juice, sip slowly.

Beets in apple cider vinegar...this makes a tasty condiment to any dish, cleanses the blood and makes a gentle, natural laxative.

Wash and peel the beets, use processor to grate, mixing with grated onions and adding any spices and seeds i.e. Nut Meg, cinnamon, caraway seeds, turmeric or curry powder etc. press down firmly and pour apple cider vinegar plus a little filtered water to just cover the beets. Place in refrigerator and use as required. If the tops are fresh, wash and freeze and use in smoothies or as a vegetable.

Heavy Metals...with the pollution all around us in this modern age it is necessary to detoxify on a regular basis.

Start the day with a cilantro and apple smoother, cilantro in known for its detoxifying effects to rid heavy metals such as mercury, lead and tin flushing them out of the body via urine and bowel movements.

Eat lots of cleansing salads and high fiber foods to assist in clearing away toxins

Nettle tea, dandelion tea and milk thistle are cleansing herbs Also drink more water to flush out the kidneys.

Many people do not drink enough water to hydrate the body.

Drinking water when you feel hungry can be exactly what you require...not always food.

A Low immune system can be caused by grief, holding on to past trauma, having someone dupe you into giving over your money, being cheated on.

The stress incurred by the situations and continuing to dwell on same can turn in to a cancer.

 Drink only distilled water (not in plastic bottles) to draw out the inorganic minerals which build up in the joints. At all other times only drink filtered or purified water

Digestive Aids

Avoid all fried foods.

Activated charcoal...good for excessive gas and stomach bugs
Bentonite clay. helpful for cleansing the colon & absorbing
stomach bugs.
Both the above require insoluble fiber and plenty of water to flush
it through the body

Probiotics are organisms such as bacteria or yeast
that research states can maintain/improve health. They can be
found in manufactured supplement in many health stores online &
on main street. They are also prolific in many natural foods.

Within the digestive system live over 500 different types of
bacteria, which maintain healthy intestines and aid food digesting
while helping the immune system to fight many infections &
viruses .

To retain good health the digestion and elimination systems need
to be working to the best of their ability.
To have good digestion your gut has to be healthy, it may be
necessary to take a probiotic supplement on a daily basis

It is important to keep the body hydrated with fluids (this can come
from fruit, vegetables and water. Be careful with fruit juices as
these have a high sugar content with no fiber to slow the sugar
down.

Having a glass of water 30 minutes before a meal will hydrate
your body so you have no need to drink during your meal. Room
temperature water is easier on the body.

Raw food provides enzymes which helps digestion, that is why it is good to start a meal with salad with minimum dressing, a little helps to absorb the vitamins.

Overcooked food has less nutrition than less cooked food. Raw food has the most nutrition except in a few cases e.g. Tomatoes and carrots. If possible eat half raw food and half cooked Try to mix the colors of vegetables to get an assortment of vitamins and minerals

Acupuncture is an ancient Chinese Japanese for of relief from muscle & joint pain. It uses sterilized needles placed in the bodies meridians to increase blood flow & relieve pain. It also claims to aid & heal many health issues such as frozen shoulder ect. Find a reliable practitioner & discuss your symptoms.

Chiropractor. has become more mainstream in recent years & can be beneficial for all types of back & joint pain that requires realignment As with acupuncture, do your own research and then find a reliable local practitioner.

Massage

The benefits of massage are well know so there is little need to go into detail. Find a good therapist that understand pressure points, lymph gland locations & is in tune with your body while doing the message. Avoid a therapist who is just doing a job for the money and find one who is dedicated to bringing relaxation, muscle tension release & joy to your body and mind.

Aromatherapy

Aromatherapy oils are fragrant and natural ingredients found in herbs, plants, flowers and fruits. Essential oils give the aroma of the plant, flower or peel and they contain dozens of complex chemicals that seem to do everything from beautifying skin or speeding up healing, to aiding in sleep to numbing headaches. When you use aromatherapy oils they are highly concentrated so only one or two drops are required. Although a small 10 ml bottle might appear expensive, it lasts a long time when kept in a cool dark place. Use caution when buying that they have been correctly stored away from heat and light. Do not confuse aromatherapy oil with a fragrance oil, which is man made from artificial chemicals and holds the smell far longer than aromatherapy oils, which evaporate in the air. Most perfumes are made up of fragrances which makes them very potent, sometimes too strong.

WARNING if you suffer from asthma or have a history of serious breathing problems or any other medical condition that can be effected by a strong aroma, do not use essential oils without first consulting your doctor.

Since the beginning of time plants have been used for food and medicine being found out by trial and error which plants were good and which ones were poisonous. The Egyptians in 4500 BC used myrrh and cedar wood oils for embalming, 6500 years later preserved mummies are proof of their skills. Modern research shows that cedar wood contains a natural fixative and myrrh has strong, antiseptic agents, which explains why most mummies look so good for their age. The Egyptians were the first to distil plants in order to extract their essential oils.

The Romans on the other hand used essential oils for giving pleasure as much as for curing pain, and had leisurely, perfumed baths and massages every day. In Greece, India, China and Arabia the use of aromatics thrived. But is wasn't until the 12 the century that perfumery and herbalist spread to Europe. By the time of the great plague in 1665 it was so well established that Londoners burnt bunches of lavender, cedar and cypress in the streets and carried posies of the same herbs as their only defense against infectious disease. Modern aromatherapy was first used 65 years ago by a French chemist. One day he was working in the laboratory and badly burnt his hand and plunged it into a vat of lavender essential oil, when his hand healed quickly without blistering, he then began his lifelong obsession - studying the therapeutic properties of plant oils.

Biochemists have recently isolated dozens of ingredients in essential oils that account for the amazing properties they have. Now that the folk remedies have been substantiated by scientific fact, aromatherapy has become widely accepted and more popular than ever before.

There are many oils which can be used alone or a combination of several oils which compliment each other. A carrier oil, avocado, jojoba, almond oil, primrose etc are used as the base adding a couple of drops of several different oils, which compliment each other. Usually 8-10 drops to 10 ml. Bottle. Do not use too much as they are very potent and requires 24 hours before using it again, just like pharmaceutical products, you would not take one days pills in one go.

Some oils soothe jaded nerves.... Chamomile, bergamot, geranium, jasmine, lemongrass.

Some oils are stimulating...peppermint, eucalyptus, ginger

Aromatherapy oils have many uses

Baths...add 8-10 drops of choice to a tub with Epsom salts and sea salt and lay back and relax. The heat and steam together with the salts and aroma will give you the finest spa treatment in your own bathroom.

Room vaporizers...ring burners which fit on lamps with 3 drops of oil, the heat from the bulb disperses the aroma, or a small pot of water on a radiator with 3 drops of oil.

Beauty treatments...personalize your beauty products, some oils rejuvenate mature completions, others reduce oiliness and they all smell divine. Cleansers, masks and moisturizers. They uplift your spirits at the same time as beautifying your skin

Footbaths...take a bowl large enough to put your feet covered in water.

Fill the bowl with comfortably hot water and use 4 drops of pine and 4 drops of eucalyptus for a therapeutic foot bath. In a relaxing bath you could use 3 drops chamomile and 3 drops of lavender.

Room sprays... Mix several drops of oil in water in a spray bottle. Shake well and spray around the room.

Air purifier...put several drops of oil in the vacuum, where the air is blown out,

Peppermint or eucalyptus

Household cleanser...add a few drops to a small bowl of water and use this with your wash cloth to wipe surfaces and clean the kitchens and bathrooms

Closets...a few drops on a cotton wool ball in a closed closet will refresh.

Bedtime...a few drops of chamomile or lavender on a cotton wool ball next to the bed to help you to relax into a deep sleep.

Coughs and colds...inhale the steam from hot water and a few drops of Olbas or eucalyptus. Also 2 drops on a handkerchief for inhaling during the day.

Hair care... good for dandruff or dull lifeless hair. Mix with a mild shampoo or mix with olive oil, a tablespoon of unpasteurized apple cider vinaigrette and several drops of cedar wood, eucalyptus or tea tree oil. Leave on the hair for 20 minutes, shampoo as usual. If you use the olive oil and apple cider vinaigrette on a regular basis and reduce your sugar intake you will be amazed at the results of your hair. Sugary foods damage the whole body and are very aging.

All essential oils are multi-purpose, the following is a limited review which each one can do. Always test on a patch of skin to check if you are allergic, people with very sensitive skin be very cautious.

A few of the most popular essential oils and their uses, many oils are multi-tasters giving choices to the aroma you like the best.

Aniseed, fennel, caraway...improves the digestive system.

Bergamot...this oil is photo toxic, do not use before going into the sun. It has many uses, it is uplifting, soothes skin conditions such as eczema, psoriasis, especially where stress or depression are a factor.

Chamomile...insomnia, stress, tension.

Citronella... Neuralgia, headaches, insect repellent

Clove ...strong antiseptic, useful in emergencies for toothache as it works as a local analgesic. (Do not use for any length of time on the gums)

Eucalyptus...strong anti-viral, bacterial antiseptic which is perfect for colds, and useful for aching muscles as it is an effective painkiller

Frankincense...used in perfumery and can be used in facial preparations, as it has rejuvenating properties, is also calming

Lavender...the most versatile of all oils. A stimulant of cell growth, treats burns, soothing, relaxing, reduces inflammation, balances emotional extremes of stress.

Lemongrass...a strong antiseptic and bactericide, acts as a sedative on the nervous system, eases muscular aches and pains she mixed with rosemary.

Mimosa...cheering, anti-depressant.

Neroli...one of the strongest stress relieving oils also rejuvenates the skin

Patchouli...this is one of a few which improve with age, regenerates skin cells, is anti fungal and has an anti-Depressant action.

Peppermint...a multi purpose oil, invigorating, energizing, good for relieving congestion, useful when mental clarity is required. Do not use in the evening.

Rose geranium...insect repellent, regulates hormone imbalances, thus has a calming effect, is excellent in skin preparations.

Rosemary...mental fatigue, headache, muscular rub to prevent muscular strain.

Sage...helps prevent sweating

Sandlewood...strong antiseptic action, can be applied to chest and throat .has a soothing effect on dry, sore or inflamed skin. Sensual, sedative

Clary sage...PMT

Spearmint...less harsh than peppermint...is a digestion aid and relieves gas [flatulence]

Yang Ylang... slows rapid breathing, soothing, relaxing anti-depressant effect.

When using the oils for a massage do not bathe or shower for at least 2 hours, allowing the oils to be absorbed into the skin

If you are deep thinker, worrying and anxious try a scalp massage.

Combine any or all of these with sweet almond oil:

Bergamot, jasmine, lavender, neroli, orange, rose.

Before you start put on your favorite relaxing music.

This massage you can give to yourself, whilst stretching your neck side to side, then leaning forward, massaging with the mixed oils, using stroking and circular movements with your fingertips, massage all over your neck, around the ear and forehead, whilst deep breathing, repeat several times from the nape of the neck to the forehead.

When you have massaged every inch, take a tiny section of hair and tug several times, repeat this with all your hair.

This will stimulate the circulation and relax the scalp. Move on to the brows, squeezing between thumb and finger along the brow, then make circular movements over the facial contours, pressing down for the count of 10 before moving on to the next spot.

When you have finished relax and enjoy the feeling of relief from the tensions of the day.

Supplements

As we age, we may not get the correct amount of nutrition if we do not have access to fresh foods. Supplements can help restore the bodies balance in many areas where there seems to be a deterioration due to wear and tear over the years. Too many supplements can be more harmful than taking none, so as with everything in life, balance is the key to wellbeing.

Supplements are a multi-billion dollar industry with a vast array of choices. Many drug store & supermarket supplements are low quality & can contain fillers & other ingredients that may not help maintain a healthy system & could possibly be detrimental taken over time.

On the other end of the spectrum there are companies that claim their supplements are superior & charge thee times the price of similar products on the market that are equal in quality & much cheaper. Shop around until you find the best supplier that will not rip you off & has a reliable return policy.

Here are a few brief suggestions of supplements that can help maintain a healthy body & mind. Try to void all pill supplements, choose capsules and remove the gelatin cover, putting the powder in a smoothie. If it is liquid bite off the top and swallow the liquid then throw away the gelatin cover. **If you are on medication, before taking any supplements, first discuss any product with your doctor.**

Coq10 150 mg a day are said to significantly strengthen the heart muscle, together with a diet rich in healthy nutrition.

Vitamin D many people do not get enough sunlight & may be deficient in vitamin D.

Natty powder has a large amount of vitamin k, which helps the bones absorb calcium, instead of it circulating in the veins to calcify. It is also good for osteoporosis . Natto is a fermented soybean product which is available in powder form.

Probiotics are necessary to maintain healthy intestines and bowels. They replace harmful bacteria with protective bacteria that aids digestion & aids the colon.

Ginseng complex capsules for libido, energy & lower blood pressure

Ginkgo capsules improves blood flow & aids brain function. Ginkgo and ginseng are a natural blood thinners.

Saw Palmetto capsules for prostrate health

Pygeum capsules for prostrate health

Spirulina powder, is a blue green algae full of vitamins, minerals, carotenoids & essential fatty acids

Vitamin C to help fight infection colds & flu.

Vitamin B complex aids to rid many symptoms associated with nerve system.

Grape seed beneficial for a number of cardiovascular problems.

Echinacea helps to protect against colds & flu. Helps to strengthen the immune system

Zinc tablets for libido, strength deficiency

'Mucus clear' droplets under the tongue to help rid congestion in the sinuses

Pine bark, for allergies or swelling excessively by insect bites. Being a natural product it takes longer than prescription remedies to take effect but will protect longer once it has established a place in the bodies natural protection system

Homeopathic remedies. This is a whole field of remedial learning & it is best to find a homeopathic practitioner or speak with a consultant in a health store that has a homeopathic department.

Organic v Conventional Foods.

Conventional foods have often been cross pollinated, grown with chemical fertilizers and sprayed with pesticides. Organic should be of original ancient seeds and grains and grown in regulated conditions. using foods as a cure for an illness it is essential to eat organic grown food, check them for freshness. Fresh vegetables are sweet, as they age the get more bitter by the day.

Wash all fruit in baking soda, salt or one of the special cleaners on the market.
Baking soda and salt are absorbent so will help pull off any surface dirt. Then wash thoroughly in running filtered water.

The most heavily pesticide foods are strawberries, apples, bell peppers, celery, cherries, grapes, lettuce peaches, pears, spinach and tomatoes.

Enzymes can become depleted as we age, if we eat mostly cooked food. Raw living foods, discussed later in the book, will replenish lost enzymes & has a multitude of health providing advantages.

The Immune System guards us from infection, disease and auto immune disorders. However if we eat high calorie low nutrition foods it will not be strong enough to protect the body from all the cells that are mutating into cancers, which are trying to attack us daily. To build a strong immune system we require low stress levels, vitamins, minerals, enzymes and antioxidants and phytonutrients. These can all be obtained from high nutritious foods (not from popping handfuls of pills). Hypocrites was correct when he said food is medicine.

If we continue on a path that is a slave to our taste bud's craving for high fat, sugar, salty foods etc, over time the immune system can rebel and start to attack the body rather than protect us from disease.

The way to unlock this necessary nutrition is to chew food until it is a more or less liquid. Digestive enzymes start in the mouth, awakening the enzymes in the stomach before the food is swallowed. Many people in this hectic age eat food on the run or eat and talk at the same time. This is a cause of poor digestion leading to indigestion as the food is swallowed in large pieces which are not digestible.

If you don't have time to eat slowly then use a high powered blender which in 2 minutes will purée all food to a creamy consistency. Some recipes will follow in the next chapter

 A regular blender cannot blend seeds and pineapple cores and some foods to a creamy consistency. Two of the best on the market are Blendtec and Vitamix. Research these two machines to see your preference. Check out prices on Amazon, make sure you get the full warranty which should be 7 years if you are not a commercial enterprise.

Margaret's Delicious Recipes

Soup Fit For Kings & Queens

Spending a few hours preparing an assortment of grains and beans can lead to a variety of quick and easy meals.
Choose 3/4 different types of beans: below is a good mixture.

Cranberry beans...much sweeter and more delicate in taste than common pintos or kidney beans, these beans are popular in Italian cuisine. They have a smooth texture and mild, nutty flavor. Perfect for salads, soups, stews and bean spreads.
Cooking time: 1 hour . 4 cups of water for every cup of cranberry beans. Bring to the boil, reduce heat and simmer for about 1hour.

Adzuki beans...although soaking is not necessary, soaking makes cooking time shorter. These beans are more easily digested than most beans due to a very low fat content. Slightly sweet flavor.
Cooking time: 1 - 11/2 hours. 3 cups water for every cup of Adzuki beans.

Black beans...high in magnesium and fiber. Very low in fat. Rich earthy flavor.
Cooking time: 1 - 1 1/2 hours3 cups of water to 1 cup of beans.

Garbanzo beans: also known as chickpeas.
Cooking time: 1 - 2 hrs. 4 cups of water to 1 cup of beans.

Soak beans in large glass jars. Fill jars with 1 cup of beans and fill up with water in the morning, in the evening pour off water, rinse and leave overnight to sprout. (This cuts cooking time down). The age of the beans makes a difference in the cooking time, if they are recently dried they cook quicker, if they are 1 or 2 years older they need a longer cooking time. although dried beans can last indefinitely the fresher they are, the better they taste. The cooking times are approximate.

To add extra flavor add a selection of diced vegetables, carrots , onions and celery.

Choose different condiments for different beans, for example: Toasted coriander , cumin and cardamom seeds whole. (Roast by heating a heavy bottomed saucepan, first put in coriander (this only takes a few minutes and requires full attention), then the cardamom and finally the cumin, which cooks in seconds.) roasting gives a different flavor.   These can be ground in a coffee grinder or left whole.

If possible cook all the beans at the same time. When cooked spoon the beans with a little juice into muffin tins, you can mix the beans or leave them separate. Once in the tins put in freezer until frozen. Remove from muffin tins and put into freezer bags. Can be kept for up to 6 months. With being in small amounts they will thaw quicker and it is easier for portion control

Original deli chopped liver Not recommended

Liver
Chopped egg
Fried onions
Chicken fat
Salt and pepper

Vegetarian Chopped liver

Sautéed onions
Cooked green beans,
Lightly toasted walnuts or pine nuts
A little olive oil
Seasoning to taste
Cut pita beads into quarters and toast.
Alternative to beans....peas
Yummy

Pesto alternative
Chop raw kale or spinach in food processor
Add chopped toasted walnuts
Chopped onion and garlic optional
Olive oil
Serve over pasta

Coconut, coconut oil

Use coconut oil for all your cooking and baking needs, use it in
place of butter.
Make sure it is organic unrefined, if it does not taste too good it is
old. Coconut oil can withstand higher heat. According to medical
research including coconut oil to you every day foods can reverse
hypothyroid gland problems. Coconut oil can increase calorie
burning by 50%, contains medium chain triglycerides, a type of
fatty acid that is easier to digest, stimulates the body's metabolism
and restores some of the body's natural enzyme activities that are
needed to maintain a healthy weight. (All raw sprouted foods are
loaded with enzymes). substitute coconut oil to replace butter.

Kale salad

Chop kale and garlic in food processor
Chop salad into small pieces (or use processor)
Chop figs and dates into small pieces
Mix together with dressing
Let marinate for 2 hours. (Will keep for 3 days)
Toast sliced almonds or walnuts and add when serving
Dry roast sesame seeds in pan and sprinkle on top

Make a grain and beans...in the last 15 minutes of cooking the beans add well washed quinoa or millet. Leave in pan with lid on for 10 - 15 minutes. Fluff with fork...serve.
This also can be used for 3 days (or freeze any extra for another day)
To make this into a different dish add chopped onions, chopped celery and cubed butternut squash (or sweet potato or cooked carrots, or both)

Dressing
Any or all of the following
Virgin olive oil,
Toasted or regular cold pressed sesame oil
Balsamic and apple cider vinegar (unpasteurized)
Soy sauce
Honey
Five spice seasoning
Turmeric
Ginger powdered or fresh grated

Using different grains, beans, vegetables, salads and other favorite dressing will give this salad a variety of tastes.

Salad....onions...radish...cucumber...celery....grated carrot
If using tomatoes add when serving

Sandwich or Cracker Toppings.

Oatmeal pita bread, cut in quarters and toasted make good crackers.

Vegetarian chopped liver

Cook any of the following dried beans and purée with onions, garlic and herbs
White beans
Garbanzo beans
Green split peas
Frozen peas
Sprouted lentils
Sprouted mung beans
Cooked sweet potato (use this instead of butter)
Avocado

Serve with mixed salad

Danish bread ...mix in the pan you are going to cook it in

1 cup organic non-irradiated sunflower seeds
half cup flax seeds
Half cup walnuts
1 and half cup rolled oats
2 tablespoons chia seeds
4 tablespoons psyllium husks or
  3 teaspoons if powder
Half teaspoon salt
1 tablespoons spoon maple syrup
  (Alternative, black strap molasses and or barley malt)
3 tablespoons coconut oil (make sure it is fresh)
1 and half cups water

Whisk maple syrup oil and water together...soak 2 - 20 hours
Preheat over to 350 degrees
Place pan on rack for 40 minutes, remove from pan and bake
further 20 minutes. Remove and place on wire rack

Tasty tofu

One packet extra firm (for a texture similar to chicken freeze until ready to use, remove from freezer and defrost in refrigerator for 2 days. Squeeze as much water out as possible before using)
Cut into small cubes and place in a Pyrex dish which has a lid
Marinate with soy sauce,
Curry powder to your taste
Dried herbs
Dry powdered garlic
Whole garlic,minimal olive oil and chopped herbs**
1 whole onion finely chopped
3-4 chopped celery stalks
Place in the bowl, put lid on and shake
Place in refrigerator until ready to use
To cook
Place on baking sheet.
A toaster oven is useful to cook this. Twice baking on the toaster control. Three times if you want it very well done.

Mixed herb dressing
*when herbs are plentiful ,basil, parsley, mint, coriander and any other herbs you like, put in food processor with garlic and chop fine. Place in glass bottles with a little balsamic vinegar and top up with extra virgin olive oil. This makes a good condiment and cooking aid for many dishes.
Keep in refrigerator for up to 9 months. Coriander, cumin and cardamom seeds can be added to give more flavor.

Side dishes

Cabbage, celery, carrots and unsweetened desiccated coconut.
Slice cabbage, onions, carrots and celery in food processor
Sauté cabbage for five minutes, add celery carrots and coconut and enough water to cover.
Simmer until cooked. Put leftovers in glass jar with screw lid for next day

Fish Patties For Two (fresh or canned cod, salmon or tuna.)

Approx 12 ozs fish of your choice
1 cup old fashioned oats (blend until finely chopped, a few seconds)
1/2 onion, (sweet, red or cooking onion)
2 sticks celery,
A few sprigs of parsley
1 teaspoon mild curry powder
2 cloves garlic
1 egg optional(gives a different flavor)

Chop the above items and place in food processor using only half the oats until blended, add more oats if necessary to make a good consistency.

Mix together remaining oats, unsweetened desiccated coconut, (chili peppers, salt and pepper. Optional)

Make into patties and dip into oat powder and cover all over.
Spray a baking tray with olive oil and sprinkle with the oat powder (this extra sprinkling stops it from sticking.)
Spray top of patties with olive oil (optional)
Bake in toaster over one and a half times on toast or cook in regular over at 375 for 15 - 20 minutes. Test for doneness.

Serve hot or cold

Steamed Salmon & Vegetables

Ingredients
Salmon, cod or trout
Cabbage leaves
Assortment of fresh vegetables
Steam of 10 minutes...check for doneness
Raw sesame oil
Lime juice
Cilantro
Sea salt
Toasted sesame seed (to toast place one tablespoon of seeds into heavy base pan on high heat,
Toast for a few seconds

Place a couple of cabbage leaves in the bottom steamer, wrap dill around the salmon and place on the cabbage leaves. On the top layer place an assortment of fresh vegetables: broccoli ,
Cauliflower, sliced peppers, asparagus, onion
SAUCE...combine raw sesame oil, lime juice and brown rice vinegar, cilantro, sea salt
When everything is cooked drizzle with sauce.
Sprinkle with toasted sesame seeds.

Yummy Deserts

Margaret's Chocolate Nut Cookies

2 bars Lindt dark chocolate
2 cops Cheerios
1 cup toasted almonds
1 cup toasted pecans
(Chop nuts and mix together)
Sugar free desiccated coconut
1 cup mixed raisins and craisins.
Cinnamon and ginger...optional
Ground chia seeds, flax seeds, hemp. (This adds 3-6-9 omega oils,
makes the cookie more filling)

To make

Melt chocolate in Bain Marie (or use a s/s bowl inside a saucepan
which has boiling water) keep the heat low.
Break chocolate into small pieces in the bowl, stirring until melted.
Remove dish, and if large enough add Cheerios. If not pour
chocolate into a larger dish.
Sprinkle in flavoring and stir to mix.
Lastly add nuts and fruit and mix altogether.
Place tin foil onto a baking sheet that will fit in the refrigerator.
Spoon the mixture onto the tray and place in refrigerator.
When set place in zip lock bag and store in fridge.

Margaret's Special Cookies.

3 cups whole oats
1 grated carrot
1 grated zucchini
1 grated Apple
(could also interchange with grated sweet potato or pumpkin (can be canned)

3 ripe bananas (or 3 thawed bananas)
(2 eggs...if you eat eggs)
Unsulphered apricots, dates figs, prunes, raisins, craisins
Almonds, walnuts (best for heart health) pecans, macadamias
Grind together flax seeds, wheat germ, poppy seed*, sesame seeds, (use any or all the above)
2 tablespoons coconut oil
1 - 2 tablespoon barley malt, ***
1- 2 tablespoons Blackstrap molasses ***
Powdered ginger
Cinnamon, nutmeg or cloves 1 teaspoon in all.

Make first batch with. 1 tablespoon and adjust to your taste when next baking them.
*obviously, leave out anything you do not like, and add anything you prefer.

In food processor add 1 cup of oats, apricots, dates and figs, and using the pause button chop. Place in large bowl
In food processor place the bananas, barley malt and black strap molasses and coconut oil, mix.
Place all the ingredients in the large bowl and mix together.
chop the remaining fine or coarse as preferred
If the mixture is too dry add more water or banana.
If the mixture is too wet add more oats.
Lightly grease a large baking tray, scatter sesame seeds and/or

unsweetened desiccated coconut. Put the mixture in blobs on the tray and smooth with a plastic spatula. Spread sesame seeds and/or coconut on top and press into the mixture so they do not fall off when baked. With a plastic spatula mark out lines the size you wish the cookies to be.

Place in centre of oven at 350 degrees and cook for 40 minutes, depending on the thickness of your cookies, usually half an inch.

Place on wire tray to cool.

If you have surplus these can be frozen, put in a toaster oven to reheat, they taste even better.

Margaret's Coconut, Oat, & Fruit Cookies

2 cups coconut flour
2 cups organic oats - grind in blender for 5 - 10 seconds if you like
it fine, or use whole
2 peeled and chopped apples, any kind.
2 ripe bananas
1 cup mixed, slightly roasted nuts, walnuts, almonds and pecans,
chopped
1/2 to 1 cop raisins and cranberries
Figs and dates...optional 2-5 of each chopped depending on taste
  The ingredients make this a sweet cookie.....no need to add extra
sweetener
Eggs...optional

Using a plastic blade
Blend bananas and eggs with 1 cup of filtered water in food
processor, add figs and dates.
Add coconut flour and oats. Add more water as necessary.
Add apples, raisins and cranberries. Mix to a smooth consistency
(Coconut flour requires more water than regular flour)
Prepare a cookie sheet, lightly grease with coconut oil, (if you do
not have coconut oil use your favorite cooking oil) sprinkle
desiccated coconut and sliced almonds on tray, optional.
Either spread mixture on sheet, spreading out with a spatula and
mark in squares or
Roll into portion controlled balls first dipping in desiccated
coconut and/or sliced almonds .
Cook for 20 minutes on 375 F for 20 minutes, check for
doneness...cook a little longer if not cooked.
These can be frozen and reheated in toaster oven another day.

Smoothie Recipes

Breakfast is the most important meal of the day, which is why they say; eat breakfast like a kind, lunch like a prince and dinner like a pauper. One of the best breakfasts is to soak oats & almond overnight then add a banana and a pear. put tem in your blender and in a minute you'll have a nutritious breakfast that will sustain you until lunch.

Here is a list on 10 smoothies that will make you feel lighter and cleansed. Use distilled, filtered water for smoothies.

1/ cabbage, broccoli stem, beets, apple, cilantro

2/ Pineapple, Kale, Mint

3/ Wheatgrass, Parsley, Apple

4 /Watercress, Apple , Mint

5/ Cucumber, Celery, Apple.

6/ Pineapple, Kale and Mint.

7/ Wheatgrass, parsley, Apple and pineapple .

8/ Watermelon with Strawberries.

9/ Lettuce, Celery, Apple and cucumber

10/ Use any 4 items for a smoothie from the list below to give a variety of flavors. Use Cilantro in all of the smoothies

Apple, Avocado, Strawberry, Ginger, Lime, Parsley, Oregano, Thyme, Lime, Pineapple, Pear, Blueberries, Raspberries, Nuts, Banana, Peach, Mango

IMPORTANT MAINTENANCE INFORMATION FOR DETOXIFIYING & KEEPING HEALTHY VIA DIET.

Sprouting Seeds, Nuts and Grains.

Now we come to the main thrust of eating healthy foods to maintain true wellness throughout our life. The following ingredients & recipe is used at many expensive spas & alterative health retreats.

It can cost $10,000 a week at a top spa or retreat to learn how to eat to regain health & cure many ways people neglect their bodies with past junk food binges.

The knowledge of wise foods you are about to read should become your main way to detoxify the system and get to the desired weight your body needs to live a life of joyful pursuits.

Your Daily Fix; Sprouted Organic Living Foods

Only do small portions of the following as it is easy to make too much.

Always use glass containers not plastic for sprouting.

Use a few of the following ingredients, and vary it each time you make it so you get the benefits of a wide range of products or even add a few of your own ideas.

All ingredients should be organic, if a seed does not sprout after 2 days it probably has been irradiated, as they now do with most organic almonds, and they do not have to mark it on the product.

Everything can be purchased at good health food stores or online via the internet. Best to buy small quantities to begin and then when you get the correct mix that suits your system buy in bulk & save money.

Sprouted bean smoothie for increased nutrients

Mung beans

Lentils

French lentils

Garbanzo beans

Sunflower seeds

Pumpkin seeds...

for starters use half teaspoon of each then adjust as you become an expert.

Mung beans, garbanzo beans and lentils can be soaked in the same container. In the morning using filtered water cover the beans with enough water to allow them to swell... drain and rinse in the evening and leave to sprout overnight, if you make too many, rinse twice a day and use the next day

Pumpkin and sunflower seeds can be soaked together, soak in the evening, rinse in the morning and use straight away.

Almond and walnuts...about 12... soak the nuts together

Flax seeds

Chia seeds

Hemp seeds

Raw buckwheat...
These four can be placed in one jar.
Half teaspoon of each,

Fill with water at night and use the next day without rinsing

Blend with any of the following ingredients to make a tasty nutritious meal.

Apple

Pear

Blueberries,

Raspberries

Blackberries

Banana

kale or mixed greens

Lettuce

Cucumber

Celery

Organic oat flakes

Almonds

Figs. *

Dates. *

Prunes. *

Avocado*

Optional . *.

*leave out if you are using the smoothie to lose weight or recover from an illness.

Use filtered water for your desired consistency

A dash of turmeric to alleviate any aches and pains...if necessary.
Put in blender with pure water, blend until smooth.
A vita mix blender or other high speed blenders are a good investment if you decide to include this drink into your lifestyle.

Once we loose weight, we can have this drink for breakfast and occasionally in the evening if we have over eaten for a few days.

It really is a miraculous way of nourishing the body.

If you make more than you need at one go, store in fridge for up to 3 days

All sprouted seeds contain probiotics so it ferments and maybe looks spongy on top the next day, this is perfectly normal, just shake the bottle or re-blend.

If you are on any medication, check with your doctor before making any changes to diet.

When soaking seeds for sprouting you can use drinking glasses or collect glass jars from products you use. It is preferable not to use plastic as it may turn food toxic over time? so I stick to glass.

Any amount of water is okay, more rather than less, as the seed soaks up the water they enlarge, as you will see after the first time and each day they sprout they just keep on doubling.

To slow the sprouting process just pop them in the fridge. They keep several days, after 3 days they are not so sweet.

Also use the sprouts on salads, or mix in with vegetables .

These sprouts are high in enzymes, as well as vitamins and minerals, when cooking food it depletes the enzymes.

Flax, chia, hemp and buckwheat go a little slimy, so you are unable to rinse these, any surplus water can be drained off.

Can be used on top of porridge oats.

In Canada they have a product containing all these seeds and they have named it Holy Crap. It makes a very good natural laxative that is not harmful.

After rinsing and placing all the ingredients in the blender fill the water about 1 inch over the contents. If it is too thick add more water. It all depends whether one likes a thick or thinner consistently.

When adding avocado it goes thick and creamy, if you put a lot of frozen fruit in it can be like ice cream.

However you like it... it is the right way.

Have fun, experiment, change it around to keep it interesting. All my recipes turn out different each time as I don't measure anything and sometimes I miss an ingredient out and have impulses to add something else.

If you use a lot of green leaves and its a little bitter add more bananas or frozen berries.

Happy Sprouting

Miracles happen every day in different ways. You can change
your health around by prayer, changing your attitude to life, eating
foods that give a strong internal army the power to overcome your
illness and commit to avoid all foods that weaken the system.
Be happy... Smile Often

Cooking With Love

If you love what you are doing and you use good quality, fresh
food it will all taste delicious.
Some people love a lot of seasoning,
Some not so much.
Some people love lots of variety.
Some people love just a few.
Some people love it well done.
Some love it rare.

When cooking you need to be adaptable. If you think a recipe has
too many ingredients, just pick out your favorites. Trial and error
makes for your perfect recipe. Even if the exact same ingredients
are used, it can turn out different each time. So just have fun and
mix a little of this, that and the other. It's amusing when people
say they cannot cook...the truth of it is they do not wish to cook.

A specific organs health is influenced by the overall health of the
entire body. Medications mostly treat symptoms, when in fact we
need to think and eat to nourish the whole body to keep it running
smoothly.

If you put gas in your car and omit to check the oil or tires, then
one day it will not be running smoothly, so it is with our body. If
we think mostly toxic thoughts, eat toxic foods then down the line
you will not get the mileage out of your body, it will start to break
down and will require drastic changes to get it back on the road.

Although today's medications are necessary to keep many alive it
is best to seek cause & effect...the secret is to change your thoughts
and diet to include healing thoughts and healing foods...and as you
start to heal you can lower and eventually stop taking medications
by working with you doctor to this end. There are many doctors
who now work with patients to change their eating habits.

Keep it Simple

Remove clutter

Good posture

Clean thoughts

Plain natural foods

Exercise and deep breathing

Live simple...stay close to Mother Nature

Weak people find weak excuses in order to continue their bad habits

I want...a strong healthy body and mind

I want...true happiness.

The information on food in the first part of the book is to help you get onto the healthy path before your body has a breakdown, thus avoiding the inconveniences of being incapacitated.

We are part of the air we breathe,
the water we drink
the sky we see,
the flowers we smell,
we all belong,
we are one,
one is all.

One Last Reminder.

No matter how healthy a diet maybe, if we suffer from mental anguish & stress while eating, the food will turn toxic while it is being digested. Stress is created by eating on the run Foods you are unable to digest fully, eating whilst anxious not chewing the food fully, arguing or controversial conversation at the table, past bad memories; etc.

When having a meal take the time to sit at a table. Take time to smell your food before eating, this helps your digestive juices to start working.

The tip of the tongue is where the taste buds reside so the more time spent chewing the more flavor you acquire, digestive juices in the tongue start the first phase of digestion making it easier for the stomach to digest the liquid matter you swallow (all food should be liquid when you swallow it.

Chew at least 30 times, if you have mindfulness when eating this will become one of your good habits when eating... It allows food to be swallowed slower, therefore you can feel when you have eaten enough food.

Eating quickly does not get the digestive juices working adequately, you swallow before the stomach has worked up enough digestive juices and this can lead to discomfort after you have finished eating.

It is preferable not to have conversation when eating, this can lead to a stomach with too much gas because the food has not been chewed enough and swallowed too quickly. Take delight in your meals and enjoy with plenty of love and Joy as the relish.

PART TWO

THINK WELL

The way we process & interpret our thoughts makes all the differences on the results we achieve in every facet of our lives.

The big question is who is it inside our head that makes our decisions and how reliable is the information it projects to live an authentic life?

The following part of the book will provide you with answers & choices you may never have thought about.

Understand, if you feel a little uncomfortable reading any essay in this section, that is a good sign something is stirring inside your head.

Keep on reading & go over anything you need to be clear about.

What The Heart Desires

The first humans on earth were a very wise race of beings. They advanced through all manner of obstacles, adversities and dangers because they were in-tune with nature and instinctively knew what was good for their body's nourishment. Had they not been so skilled in survival and enjoyment of life, the human species would never have weathered the torrential storms of evolution.

As time progressed humans became intellectuals and scorned natures wisdom. Accordingly, most humans today associate themselves as a race of well educated intellectual/Ego Beings.... Nature's wisdom is in very short supply, but no matter... A "good education" is far more important than true insights. Society has an abundance of educated professors, doctors, clergy, etc., and more mayhem and wars than ever before. Where is the sense and logic to that? The ancientness of the human species is blowing in the dust, whilst its descendants continue to sink deeper, into the intellectuals/egos/(devils) merciless clutches.

Every human doctrine has just enough sprinkling of truth in it to sustain its supporters in gratifying ignorance ... They will argue and fight to uphold their intellectual teachings at the sacrifice of universal intelligence. The tinge of truth contained in their doctrines will be sufficient to allow the rest of the mind to be congested with outrageous non-sense within man made symbols, labels and dogma.

Truth Transcends ... *conjecture, doubt, speculation, presumptions, thesis, suppositions, gamble, theory, assumptions, protocol, formality, ritual, dogma, atheism, religion, ologys and all isums.*

So why should humanity settle for anything less than...The Truth? What's that you say...who knows the truth? Just ask your heart... For it cannot lie. When it is maltreated and abused... it will stop working... and the truth will always prevail. Each individual mortal being has the ability to live a carefree, wholesome, healthy, prosperous life. All mortals have trillions of cells coded to understands and reproduce in a perfect, natural system.

The heart, lungs, spleen, kidneys, liver, etc., all know how to perform their tasks in a flawless synchronicity with all of earth's generous bounty. Humanities macrocosm is governed by Nature, Universe, God, Cosmos ...These are all names/labels that describe the same manifestations in human terminology.

All are clearly visible to the wise, knowing, aware "naked" minds eye. Being in-tune with nature means being in-tune with bodily requirements, which maintain its perfect creation/evolving blueprint. The conscious mind and memory can and does lie to the body, but the body cannot lie to the mind. The body will rebel if it is maltreated and addictions and falsehoods will destroy a body well before its shelf life is up.

Here are just a couple of examples of the egos ignorance out of thousands I continue to encounter... I was invited to a fancy party at the local yacht club recently. A very charming couple, to whom I am acquainted, proceeded towards me and we began to talk. Whilst we were talking, the man ordered two large double Vodka's. He then went to the snacks table to fill his plate with crackers that contain trans-fats and a variety of cheeses that produce mucus.

Whilst he was away filling his palate, his wife told me they are having a bad time of it, as her husband is receiving treatment for prostate cancer. Chemotherapy, radiation, medication were all helping him to recover from all the damage he had inflicted upon himself.. And how was he helping himself? ...Two double Vodkas and dairy products with crackers that contain hydrogenated fats? A few moths later he died from his symptoms.

The meal served to everyone in the room (most whom are elderly and on medications) was prime rib steak with butter creamed potatoes. The desert was high fat ice cream with added cream, a highly hydrogenated fat cookie, all topped off with butterscotch source. Another person who was on my table was in a hospital cardiac ward two days earlier. He asked for an extra serving of dessert. (Do you know anyone like this?)

When the brains mis-conditioned taste buds rule the mind and body, the heart is incapable of passing its messages of love and joy until it is too late. It will eventually react to its ill treatment, but alas, many times ... it is a terminal performance.

The messages from our hearts desires may exist outside of our intellects comprehension, but it is within our intelligence's awareness. Therefore: if we cannot give our bodies the nourishment and exercise it desires (with all the knowledge and information science provides) to keep healthy and strong....

1. What chance do we have in keeping our minds (which have a very complex mechanism for administering, truth, wisdom and love) clear of worry and anxiety?

2. If we cannot manage our own health and mental emotional condition, what chance do we stand in guiding our families and work colleagues?

3. What chance do we stand to captain a ship (find true prosperity) if we cannot steer our own lives in the correct direction?

We do not need to gamble and rely on our intellect/egos version of truth. We just require a little time to listen in silence to the hearts intelligent desires. To listen in quietude to authentic meaning... To listen to the appeal from the heart... To listen to a source of truth that cannot lie.

Once we comprehend the hearts truth, we can begin to progress and live an authentic life.

"Every heart that has beat strongly and cheerfully has left a hopeful impulse behind it in the world, and bettered the tradition of mankind."- Robert Louis

Oh, what a tangled web we weave, once we practice to deceive.
(The Heart) -William Shakespeare

"When Health is absent....Wisdom cannot reveal itself....Art
Cannot become manifest ... Strength cannot be exerted.....Wealth
is Useless and.....Reason is powerless" - Herophilies - 300 B.C.....
(What has changed in 2,300 years?)

The Marrow

The Frugal family always had a marrow with their meal every Sunday. Mom would take the marrow out of the fridge and cut both ends off. Then put it in the large modern oven to cook. Little daughter Sadie would watch her mum do this every week, then one day she remarked....Mum, why do you cut both ends off the marrow...

Well Sadie, my mum taught me to cook and she always cut both ends off the marrow. Oh! I see, replied Sadie.

A few weeks went by and Grandma was visiting. Whilst they were eating dinner, Sadie looked at Grandma and asked....
Why do you cut both ends off the marrow when you cook it Grandma...Well Sadie, I've always been very old fashioned and only have a small oven and it does not fit in, if I keep it whole!

Many times in life we do things out of habit and not because they make any sense.

Mastering The Recognition of Our Stupidity.

Until a person can call themselves stupid (without blaming themselves for their stupidity) an authentic life will elude them. This statement may horrify those folks who are intellectually fed and lead, however, if their intellect is not controlled by the truth and wisdom from their universal intelligence (and very few are), they will continue to fall into big holes, without ever recognizing how they are inflicting suffering on themselves.

To become a success in the game of life, we really need to learn how to become a master in the art of stupidity in an intelligent manner. We cannot overcome any form of stupidity without first recognizing and admitting we have it. Denial of stupidity will only serve stupidities erroneous purpose & give us continual problems to overcome. Understand, there are two forms of stupid.

One which I do not recommend tolerating is filled with ignorance of the fact that stupidity is part of the daily make-up and this type of person only lives by intellectual thoughts that have been handed down over thousands of years of collective rules and regulations. Their stubborn egotistical nature leads them into all types of pitfalls. For instance; if a person who deems themselves to be clever & continually eats all the wrong type of foods that are making them sick & has to take medication to relieve the symptoms of their stupid eating, is that clever or stupid?

The other type of stupidity which I do subscribe to is… not buying into ones own smartness and questioning all A-ctions, T-houghts, C-leverness, before they ACT.

Because I have been called stupid all my life, by people who deemed themselves to be clever, I guess I can award myself the highest degree of recognizing my stupidity in every aspect of daily living.

If we cannot recognize our own stupidity then we will rely on our intellectual cleverness to work things out for us and the results will rarely produce a successful life on earth, even though society may view it as successful.

Remember, stupidity has two sides to it. One side is self evident by humanities erroneous actions and events since the beginning of cleverness without a true guiding light. This form of stupidly be-lie-ves it has mastered stupidity, yet all the results say otherwise. Therefore they have become a slave to their own stupidity and disguise it with flawed systems and policies that herd mentalities accept as normal ways to live.

The other side to stupidity is the simple mindfulness that identifies itself and thus can overrule its cleverness, so that it can make better choices. This type of stupidity has been embraced by every sage and person of wisdom since the beginning of time. In their day they were mostly executed or tortured for their so called stupidity and yet it has stood the test of time.

Most people live in an intellectual zoo locked into a cage of their own self-cleverness. Some try to attract other to join their be-lie-fs by writing a book or giving a lecture. Some may be reward for their antics with tasty morsels like awards or accolades. I suppose not too many people would be happy living in a zoo and yet so many do live locked in a mind-set of imprisonment, caught in a cage of perceptions, ideas, thoughts and suggestions (PITS). A be-lie-f system that completely overwhelms the conscious brain very rarely changes its outlook on life.

The awareness of my own stupidity allows me to live in comfortable contentment. Why not awaken to your own stupidity then you have a good chance to overcome it?

The Ten Advantages of An Awareness of Self-Stupidity

1/ We allow ourselves time for closer inspection of important decision making and restrict our ego/intellect from taking hold of the conscious mind.

2/ We do not allow our own cleverness to take us on a wild ride that may seem fruitful, yet on closer inspection we realize, the consequences of our actions may not be the outcome we desire.

3/ When other people say we are stupid we can agree with them and then they have nothing left to attack us with.

4/ Once we can acknowledge our own stupidly other peoples absurdities becomes obvious. Wise folks learn from other peoples mistakes.

5/ Forewarned is forearmed… By living in the center of our stupidly we can see the dangers that lurk before we act out our roles and thus guide ourselves on a more simple route through life's mazes…Which in turn guides us to live an amazing life.

6/ Expert advice is examined far more closely and nothing is taken for granted.

7/ By understanding our stupidity, our awareness of dangers takes on greater might and alerts us to risks more clearly.

8/ It is not only wars and conflicts that are foolhardy, it is also unnecessary risks taken in peace time such as climbing a mountain in a blizzard that bring about an early demise. People who are aware of their stupidity will not attempt to take on nature as they do not possess the ego that makes them think they are mightier than God.

9/ A person's awareness of their stupidity allows them to understand all negative emotions are illusions and thus not real. Therefore their immune system is not open to stress. However, all devious cleverness constantly seek perfection taking life seriously .Many experts who try to teach us how to mange stress, are open to the negative emotions they are trying to teach us to control. Stress cannot be managed because it stems from the illusions of the ego but it can and must be eliminated. Understand worry, fear hate etc; blocks the brain from making intelligent decisions. Dishing out strong medications that dim the senses and can induce suicide is not an acceptable answer for most people.

10/ By living out our daily awareness of stupidity in a joy filled mind, we find more success in better health, greater wealth, and abundant happiness. Also, we do not overestimate our power to change anyone. What works will prove itself and what doesn't work will testify to the clever, stupid ignorance of a misguided society.

Certainty and uncertainty wear the same mask. In hindsight we find what was true. By closer self examination of the way we process thought, we can head off many future dangers. The only way to eliminate stress is to be aware of the cause of it and if we feel it can't be eliminated because we are too clever by our understanding of managing it, We are real stupid with no signs of mastery over it. We do not want to end up our lives with the word; "Why have I been so stupid"?

Eliminating Stress, Maintaining Wellness Naturally

Who am I? Where is my place on earth? Wise sages have discussed these two questions since the beginning of human time. If these questions cannot be authentically answered and lived, then humanity will cease to exist. Without any doubt, daily world and local events, family disputes, money problems, job security, and health issues can lead to depression, fatigue and anxiety. This in turn can lead to overeating the wrong type of foods, lack of exercise, addictive habits such as smoking, alcoholic drinks and recreational and medical drugs.

You may ask how I have the answers to two of the most demanding questions ever raised. I was born with weak genes and a family history of heart attacks and cancers is not very conducive to living a long and healthy life. I realized many years ago that I cannot manage stress and if I allow stressful situations to attach to my brain I will surely succumb to an illness. Therefore, it made perfect sense to me to eliminate stress from my life.

Now, you might be thinking that is impossible to do. I agree it is impossible to do if you are a normal person that buys into everything they are told by so called experts.. Happily, I have never been accused of being normal. I am a natural person because

I identify myself as an eternal creative energy that does not rely on an ego or personality to act out my roles in this lifetime on earth. I have found that when I observe any damaging, negative thoughts such as anger or spite as the witness rather than the participant, they will evaporate before I can act them out. Let's examine five problematic areas of life that can enhance positive health and wealth. Then I will show you the secret code that will unlock your true potential to archive the five maintenance points effortlessly.

Communication with family and friends.

Changing the conversation from idle gossip and chatter to meaningful dialogue can make a difference in your life. It keeps your mind in trim order and helps every cell in the body to regenerate healthy particles. We are told that we need to socialize with other people or else we may become depressed by isolation. If we have a choice to associate with negative gossips or be alone with happy thoughts there is no contest. The best remedy is to find people who like to parley in meaningful conversations. It does not need to be boring. In fact the opposite is true. Idle chatter is boring even though it has become an addictive way of expression

At meal times ban all smart phones & other gadgets from the dinner table. Family meals together are a luxury that do not last too long. The children grow into adults fast & then they leave home to make their way in the world. Spread your wisdom when you are gathered around the table enjoying the fruits of your labor. Once the kids leave give them the space & freedom to do what they need to do without interference but always be on hand to give advice when it is asked for.

Money Matters

Is money the root of evil or a beneficial ingredient that can enhance your lifestyle. Do you feel the need for greed or do you understand when enough is enough? Do you require expert advice? Is it your money they are after or do they have the ability to genuinely help you?

Do you pay high brokerage fees? Bank fees? Insurance fees such as life, extended warranty, old age care ? Do they give you an umbrella and ask for it back when it rains? Are you in debt? The only person you can depend upon is yourself and you are about to do just that!

Overeating and Addictions

Food - junky or healthy eater? Overeating gluttony.
When the urge to overeat or needlessly snack tries to sneak up on you have you been told to fight back with these ideas?

• Put on some dance music or dance with yourself if you do not have a partner.

• Go for a walk
• have an invigorating shower
• go out to a bookstore or library
• do some sit-ups and press-ups
• If you drink - Alcohol, coffee, sodas change it to simple filtered water. Dehydration is the cause of many illnesses that lead to disease... If you have tried all this good advice and you are still addicted then you need to change something else in your life.

Exercise
Exercise can become harmful when it grows into over exertion or an addiction. Moderate exercise such as walking, swimming, yoga, stretching, and a few minutes work out with light weights is all that is required to maintain a fit body. The most important factor is to exercise the mind. I'm not sure where this quote originated however I have modified it a little and it will fit in with what you will read shortly ...

Don't walk in front of me, I may not follow. Don't walk behind me, I may not lead. Walk beside me and together we will embrace love and joy.

What can you control? Only your own emotions and perspective of what you experience through your senses. Everything passes in time, so it seems foolhardy to dwell on events that are happening at this moment in time. Pack all your woes into baggage (thoughts) that is easily disposable. Then buy into new luggage (thoughts) that only contain love and joy. They are easy to carry because they are weightless. Every new day that dawns frames your mind onto an empty canvas so you can paint a fresh picture cultivated by the cargo of love & joy. You are now about to find out how to live at the right location to address everything you care about. Firstly, read and meditate on this three line haiku for a few hours before you read the explanation that follows it.

Circle
The 361 degree
The mystics point

You are the extra one in the center of the 360-degree circle. Without your one degree there would be no circle simply because you would not exist.

Every wheel needs a hub so that it can turn with balance and precession. The hub is stationary and the wheel revolves around it. The roles you play revolve around the thoughts in your mind. You are both the activity and the motionless at the same moment in time.

Your physical form is in motion whilst your central control affects the parts that move. Your real abode is in the center of the hub with 360 spokes connected to you. Each spoke (degree) is a tree that contains the roles you play on each branch of that section of your life. a place of love, truth and beauty. At the base of the trunk of each tree is the root of truth

The branches spread segments of the truth. The blossoms are on the tip of each branch that become full of fruit (fruitful) - They contain Divine flashes of wisdom that make you healthy, wealthy and wise. Your mortal self lives on the surface of the wheel (earth) where each branch manifests into human actions fed by yearnings and desire.

You live on the rim in your human garbs. This is the place of discontent or pleasure. For most people who recognize it as their only home, it quickly fills with numerous mental catastrophes and pitfalls... It is a place where the intellect, ego and personality enjoy or endure their life on earth. In your central location, you live in a place where your intellect, ego and personality cannot influence the direction you will travel.

You become the - Self-Existent 'One.' You make great progress from this location, the more you understand it is your only real source of natural evolving creativity, that feeds the surface role-plays in the temporal space you perform them. You are infinite, you are eternal, you are a creative magnificent force in your true nameless identification.

Home is where the heart is ...
The heart of the matter is a symbol of love,
To balance the past with the future, you need to become the fulcrum of the center of the moment.
You are the small i, a fulcrum in the center of the circle of life.
The seer of intelligence, directed by the big I.
The I (invisible eye) of your creating evolver,
Some call it God, others say 'by chance.'
Whatever label you appoint, it is your only source of intelligence and creative energy.
Together you make life on earth a paradise.
A Garden of Eden that never needs to become stressed out or affected by living amongst family, friends, money, eating, addictions or anything that surfaces from unsavory minds.

Gatherings

One sunny morning, a man was walking in a park overflowing with beautiful flowers and trees. He was holding a large basket over one arm. Every so often, he would grab out at the sky and put something into his basket. A small boy was watching the man with considerable fascination. After a while, his curiosity got the better of him. He approached the man and asked, pardon me mister, but what are you doing?

The man replied, this afternoon I am to give a keynote speech at a grand historic conference. It will be attended by all the greatest minds in the world who believe in their own opinions, ideas and perceptions of the truths, in their religions and science.

I am grabbing different aspects of truth, putting them all in my basket, so that I can present them to all the noble minds. It may enable them to study and understand their own truths more clearly. The little boy looked inside the basket to find it full of thin air.

Holding a Paradise Party

Do you think it is about time you hold a paradise party? Pardon, what is that you ask, what is a paradise party? Well, a paradise party is a celebration where you invite all your nearest and dearest to celebrate life in love and joy. I am not speaking about all your acquaintances, relatives and friends. I propose you invite your real closest nearest and dearest. All your body cells, molecules, atoms and particles ... Don't you think they deserve a treat with all the punishment you have been directing their way all these years?

- All the stress, anger, fear, junk food, medications with damaging side effects.
- All the self-inflicted, polluted thoughts you have allowed to congest your brain.
- All the junk, cigarette smoke, alcohol contamination.
- All the negative people who try to wind you up ...
Especially all the close friends and relatives who can have the most influence on your psyche.

Yes, ask yourself, is it about time you hold a paradise party? You start by taking a good look at the way you are thinking. Are you expressing opinionated perceptions or are you living observational truths? If you have mastered the past, unfavorable mind conditioned stage in your life, and now negativity bounces off you like water off a ducks back, you are ready for the next stage of development.

If you are speaking authentic truths, most close-minded people will run away from you. That is a useful way to set the scene for the paradise party to begin, for it will not start without a few nips and tucks on who or what you think you currently know. There are only a few people on earth at this moment in time that knows how to hold their own paradise party. So now you want to know do you hold your paradise party?

- Your body weight should match your frame, so you are the correct weight for your build. There is no need to go on a fad diet. Just listen to your body and feed it the healthy wholesome foods and nourishment it requires, no more, no less.
- Do not drink alcoholic drinks or sodas.
- Have a smile on your face and spread love and joy to everyone you meet and greet.
- Make enough money for your requirements by giving your best efforts in every endeavor.
- Become independent of other people's opinions.
- Treat everyone with the same respect no matter whether the other person is insulting or applauding you.
- Understand a mythical fabricated God, with human traits, conditions many fears. A truer God projects love and joy, not fear and jealousy.
- The free spirit within you is an essence of intelligent energy that lifts you to higher dimensions of thought, free from prejudice and narrow-minded bigotry.

Not too many people live inside their real comfort zone. Most people you meet are conditioned with a negative slant on life through their past education and upbringing. You should understand they do not know how to change their emotional equilibrium scales and believe they are living as they choose to live. The fact they are destroying their immune system and mental balance, does not seem to matter one iota. Observe them with an objective detachment and learn from their self-destructive approach.

By not making any demands from negative minded people to accept your free mindedness, no matter who they are, you will automatically receive the inner psychological tools to help compose your mental paradise party and allow it to be celebrated with glee. ... Remember, you are, your own, one and only, guest at your minds paradise party. You live within an authentic world of your own choices, inside the recess of your mind, for the rest of your lifetime on earth.

If you are in a situation where you are being bullied you tactfully tell people that your joy-filled mind will not tolerate their insults Your frankness and honesty will turn many close-minded people away, running with their unsavory tail between their legs. They will look for some other weak character to pick on ... Someone else who is more receptive to the emotional negativity... Someone who will soak up like a sponge all their erroneous nonsense, but it will not be you anymore!

If you do not depend on anyone else for a living and can stay independent from human opinion, good, bad, or indifferent, you will become excellent in hosting your own paradise party. Your immune system and psychic will love and thrive on it.

If friends and relations try to make you feel guilty, it does not mean you try to apologize for anything you did with good intent. You do not have to make any special requests from them so that they speak to you. However, you can keep in contact, speaking to them on occasions where you meet up, transmitting love and joy to them all the time you chat. One day, someone who is now negative minded may follow your example, thank you and hold their own paradise party in synchronicity with yours ... if they don't, well, just enjoy the paradise party you are holding and expect nothing in return.

Maybe the time has yet to come before everyone else follows your paradigm. One fine day the time will come for everyone to hold a paradise party. However, that will happen if it is meant to be, at the appropriate time and place. In-between time, enjoy the pure paradise of knowing you have the intelligent universal energy, fed from up high, that will make your party swing eternally with divine bliss...Enjoy!

Why become a toxic carrier pigeon for negative thoughts other people plant in your brain, once you digest the garbage they tell you?

Replacing A Fear Forest With Inner Wisdom

A fear forest may sound a little like a title of a fictional horror story. Unfortunately, fear forests grow in most people's minds to varying degrees. The forest is better known by its scientific name of neurons & they record all our thoughts Although they grow out of illusionary thoughts, the effects can wreak real havoc in a person's life. Since nobody has ever heard of a fear forest before it would be a good idea to explain how a fear forest grows in a persons mind.

Its seeds grow very early in a baby's life. The DNA and genes of past generations can plough the fields of the mind, so that fear seeds grow easier in the mind of genes passed down from past worriers, but that is not the real reason fear forests grow. It could all depend on what developments there are in the baby's background events and how they influence the crops in their young inquisitive mind.

Will they mature radiant rosy pictures, or will the growth become dense fear forests … filled with all types of nasty negative thoughts? The habits and actions of the baby's parents are paramount and will have the most effect. If a mother or father has a tendency to worry regularly, anger quickly, or suffers from depressive mood swings, the infant will pick-up on all the fear-based behaviors.

As the neurons of the mind develop, past memories will call a group of neurons together to form a clump of memories that become negatively induced. As the child grows into adolescence and then to adulthood, more neurons that are negatively programmed lock together … The fear forest growth becomes much thicker. Whole forests of neurons cling to one another so that fear is paramount in the mind most of the time. This becomes what is known as a habitual worrier. It grows into the regular reference point in the brain of a person who becomes hooked on fear-based worries, which in turn can lead to deep depressive moods and lack of energy.

Often high fat, sugary foods are digested to try to comfort the plagued person. However, eating consoling junk foods only adds to cultivating the habitual fear forest … It weakens the immune system by lack of proper nutritious foods that feed the brain, inducing an additional lack of energy.

The worry habit enhances a vicious circle of seeing life through the continually growing fear forest, which in turn releases harmful chemicals in the body that produce adrenaline and other chemicals to fight the imaginary fear. With no foe to fight, the chemical hormones produce free radicals that attack the immune system and kill all the good cells that protect the mind and body from disease.

The mind physically grows fear by interlocking a given number of neurons programmed to react by a trepidation mentality. If this condition is only treated with psychotic drugs, the effects of the drugs may relieve or mask the symptoms short term, however, over time they may lead to more agony that is psychological.

The side effects of the drugs may induce other illness, which the body finds hard to cope with or even suicidal thoughts. Stronger drugs may be prescribed while the unbalanced person's fear forest continues to expand, veiled by the medications. So what is the answer? How does a person strike a match to burn past negative thoughts? How can they weed out all the growth of negativity that has taken a lifetime to cultivate?

What is the key to unlock the interlocked fear generating neurons?

It takes great determination from the distressed person to make a dramatic change in the way they perceive the world. The change is best accomplished by acting before the dependence on strong medications is prescribed. Prevention of mental illness is the best cure before any mental illness takes root. Therefore, a keen self-awareness of any conditioned thinking is a daily examination every person needs to resolve. They should become an observer of their own lives in a detached state of mind from a neutral location in their thoughts. Once they can become the witness of any continual negative afflictions, they need to find a quite place to relax and formulate a new living image of their brains structure.

They take a few deep breaths and then picture how the stress related thoughts are growing on their minds neurons, filled with inedible fruits that have been poisoning their system. As they view this picture, they notice interlocking branches of the tree where negative neurons have been trained to re-enforce one another.

They realize this bond needs to be broken and when it is, all infected fruits (thoughts) will cease to exist. Once the neurons untwine from each other, the fear forests weaken. The person should then both inwardly, outwardly smile, and visualize burning the smile into the joints where the neurons interlock.

They should recite meaningful, affirmative poetry or mantras, while feeling spectacular swells of pleasure drilling apart the interlocking negative neurons. Quite amazingly, the neurons will start to detach from each other and their fear forest starts to evaporate into thin air.

The fear forest does not stand any chance of survival when spiritual will power receives a divine source of wisdom that is infinite in scope and ceaseless in reach. The universal limitless power unbinds all the unfavorable fearful energy that existed in the fear forest.

They start to cultivate new glowing, succulent crops that are delectable to the taste buds of the cells in the immune system.

The whole shape of the forest changes for the welfare of the mind and body. Flourishing healing chemicals are released that aid the body's recovery system. Once again, the mind and body is reborn in balance, with the wisdom of the universe supplying daily thoughts that are productive and fertile for creativity.

Everything in the human mind's garden grows with delectable divine bliss... New outcrops of thought convey rays of sunshine on every branch of the revitalized neurons ... Not only in the mind of the rejuvenated person; it also sends intents of positive wave power towards every other person in their lives.

Some friends and family may become aware of the change and willingly choose to change their perceptions of life in the same manner.

By way of the minds intelligence system the fear forest has cut back all its illusionary fears ... In its place grows invigorated neurons, fostered by a master gardener, who planted the seeds of humanity on earth billions of years ago.

The brain, free from restrictive, anxious thoughts, performs its daily tasks with energized self-worth, vigorous self-esteem and constructive self-value.

Freedom from Fatigue Propelled Depression

The latest federal statistics in the USA, declare one in ten teenagers suffer from major depression and many use recreational drugs or alcohol to try reliving the stress. The number on prescription drugs is even higher and over one million, attempt suicide each year.

Around ten thousand succeed in their suicidal attempt. It is obvious not anyone who is fatigued can think clearly. The more stress a person is under, the more drained they feel. A downward spiral often ends in fatal devastation. Popping a pill, alcohol or cigarettes to relieve stress may be a quick fix solution for some people, but it does not take away the cause of the stress. Rather, it only masks the basic problems so that they multiply and return with greater force after the effects of the artificial stimulants dissipate.

Even well educated, happily married, athletic, physically fit, successful adults can suffer from depression and there is not a whole lot they can do about it with normal treatment. The general, so called established solutions, from medical and religious departments may not aid their plight.

A few years ago, a forty-four year old doctor, distinguished as one of the most outstanding in his field of expertise, hung himself in his garage on a sunny Sunday morning. He was receiving treatment from his own doctor, had be accepting psychiatric help, was under the support of his priest, but none could assist his afflicted, disorderly, negative mind-set.

Across the Western affluent world, there are many similar cases. Therefore, what is the answer to unlock the imprisoned minds of so many people, so that the bright light of trustworthy meaning can penetrate the doom and gloom?

Both educated and unlearned people suffer from the same complaint of depression so no amount of counseling, advice, intellectual reasoning, and logical thinking may solve the problems. If modern methods do work, why have all the people died too soon in their life from melancholic induced accidents, suicides and illness? They all perished and every moment that goes by, another person passes-on before their allotted time. So what are the alternatives that can assist a troubled mind?

• A good diet of wholesome foods, whole grains, fruit and vegetables will help.

• Extra antioxidants will aid the body to overcome nutrition-depleted foods.

• Regular exercise will improve overall health.

• Sleeping soundly throughout the night will provide clearer thoughts.
• Drinking ten glasses of water a day will help.

• Deep breathing at selected points of the day will lessen tension

• Finding time for silent time-out for five minutes, three times a day will help.

• Massage will lend a helping hand

• Mediation will quiet the mind for a while.

• Doing charitable work will take the focus off the self for a while.

However, none of the above will be a lasting solution to an ongoing basis for reoccurring issues and unpleasant circumstances in any persons life. One ageless answer will prove to be a sure - fired success in alleviating fatigue driven depression, and negative, gloomy thoughts.
A complete overhaul of self- identification is required before any person can truly bring about a change in overall well-being and happiness. A contented mind is a happy mind. It can only be

contented if it is free from thoughts and memories installed by other people's ideas, beliefs and opinions from early childhood.

If the reference points in the mind are continually playing themes that induce fear, hatred, jealousy, worry and depression, then no external aid will take that away. Only if a person realizes that all negative emotions are illusions can they tear themselves away from their egos persistent afflictions.

And, my - oh- my, what a task they have to conquer, when almost every medical professional declares negative emotions are real. When every physiologist I have come across asserts stress is real and needs to be treated directly.

What chance does any person stand when illusionary conditions are being treated by artificial academic means, which only treat the symptom and ignore the cause.

Academic thoughts, left to their own devises, will invent all manner of acceptable treatments and diets that will become the normal practice over a period of time. It is acceptable for a mind to fill with academic knowledge, but it is only of significant advantage if it is used as a tool for creative thoughts.

Creative thoughts expand the mind so that the outcome supports the individual person and humanity to grow in a continuing authentic manner. To turn fatigue depressions into vital organic thought, a change in the egos illusions of negative emotion is required ... A metamorphose into the reality of authentic love & joy is required. Thoughts that emanates from the true identity of self, inherent in every person on earth from birth. Sorry academia, but there is no substitute for the real accomplishment of trustworthy thoughtfulness, served by a seemingly empty, nonetheless, creative mind.

Every cell molecule and atom of a human being is filled with intelligent energy that conveys serene tranquility, when fed the correct thoughts.

When they are fed erroneous thoughts they rebel and formulate free radicals that destroy the mind and body, for they do not want to live in an erroneous decimating state of existence. The essence of love & joys energy fills the apparent nothingness that connects each strand of the trillions of cells in the human framework.

However because science cannot identify the empty space in each cell does not mean nothing is going on. Just the opposite is true. In the empty nothingness of every cell exists the dance of primary life that organizes a wholesome being.

When we tune into the nothingness of each cell we can rejoice with their intrinsic delight. When this realization passes through from our subconscious to our conscious mind it is impossible to feel anything other than love & joy, no matter what external circumstances are playing out their illusionary role-play.

Changing the concept of who we believe we are is the only way to dissolve depression for good.

The Joy of Truth And Wisdom.

In recent years, scientific medical studies have concentrated their focus on the effects of a joyful mind. The aim is to determine if blissfulness can maintain a person's good health and wellbeing. The studies are disclosing what wise sages have known for centuries …That a joy-filled mind will strengthen the immune systems resilience regards disease and supply all-over good health.

Even with all the new medical and spiritual information, people are less happy than previous generations. It seems the more affluent people become, the more misery they have to endure. Maybe many people surrender their joy in the expectation other people will return it to them.

• Do you live your life waiting for other people to lift your spirits?

• Are you dependant on shopping for luxury items to give you a quick fix of satisfaction?

• Do you need to be part of a social-set before you feel fulfilled in your personal self - esteem?

• Can you sit silently alone in a room, without reading a book, watching TV, talking to a friend or family member?

• Are you content and serene inside your own skin?

Many psychologists assert human beings are social animals and can develop depression if they are not part of a social group. As with most modern psychotherapy I read, I differ in my approach in overcoming the emotions of depression and unhappiness.

Being part of a social group can make demands on a person's naturalness and many times will alter their simplicity into a more unnatural sophistication. Humanity has neatly packaged itself into different groups, tribes, religions, cultures and traditions.

Most people have no choice in their conformity, because, by the time they reached seven years of age, the die-has-been-cast and their reference points established.

However, once people mature and become fully fledged members of their clans, many inner feelings of dissent and discord can fester in the subconscious mind. These uneasy feelings can last a lifetime, but the person is powerless to break away for fear of retribution from the other clan members, who are mostly sensing the same uncomfortable pressures.

Traditional habits are the most difficult to overcome, even though they may be pointless. Before I go any further, I am not advocating you should become a hermit. Rather, I am contending it may not be a good idea to allow your joy to be dependant on any outside forces.

To segregate your happiness by a reliance on any other person actions and emotions is to give up the powers of the joy you inherited at birth. Here is a small sample list of the many ways you may be segregating your joy to other people in the hopes they will return the joy with interest.

1. Are you reliant on your child's success as a substitute for what you believe to be the failures in your own life's ambitions?

2. Do you live your life through the pages of the fashion magazines always needing to keep up with the latest trends to feel worthy?

3. Are you trying to imitate your favorite film, TV or pop star, whilst longing for their fame and fortune?

4. Do you need an award or certificate to convey you are a success?

5. Are you dependent on a compliment to give you an air of self-value?

6. Do the perceptions in your faith, ideas within your spirituality or theories in your non-beliefs, contain any attached elements of fear or anxiety?

7. Are your digested, conditioned thought principles, bringing all the rewards you should expect from then ... i.e. health, wealth, comfort and happiness? If not, what useful purpose do they serve, if their performance is redundant and cannot relieve the stress of modern day living.

Throughout your life, significant circumstances will continually change for better or worse. However, the one real feeling that should grow moment by moment is your sense of joy. That can only be accomplished by a true sense of self... of who you are, and your rightful place on earth. You belong right where you are located at any given moment in time, for you are an outgrowth of universal love that has evolved and created all you see, smell, touch, see and hear.

During your lifetime, your bliss is your immortal treasure that conveys wellbeing and prosperity. Beyond all your role-plays, you are an infinite bundle of joy packaged in a human body and mind that wants to explore all things material and tangible, whilst at the same time recognizing the identity of non-tangible blissfulness. Without this recognition, life will become meaningless and the search for happiness becomes a trivial pursuit that has no real rewards.

You cannot give your bliss away; you can only conceal it from your mind with the aid of your egos perceptions. So, enjoy your family, friendships, clans, religions, spirituality and culture, but never depend on any for your authentic joy...**Your joy is full of truth and wisdom. It is who you are, within every cell and molecule of your being.**
Be at-ease with the wisdom of knowing it is time to stop playing hide and seek with your happiness. It can never leave you without your permission to hide and now you know it has nowhere to run.

Why Me!

I live on the edge of the ocean and I was looking out the window the other day. A small rainsquall hit one area of the ocean. Large white caps danced in tormented rage as the black cloud hung over that small section of water. It made a perfect circle and all around the squall was relatively calm water with no white caps.

The section of the ocean being pummeled may have thought – Why me? – What have I done to deserve being tossed around like this? Why is this black cloud hang over me whilst all around me is bathed in sunshine?

Ocean can't talk human language, but if it could, I'm sure that would have been its feelings.

Nearly every person on earth will be hit by squalls of anguish at some point in their lives. Seemingly random actions of doom and gloom will come into their lives from out of the clear blue sky and they will look up and say "Why me?

On the surface, there is no real reason why anyone is singled out for random chaos. There are many reasons why people bring on their own bad health, finance, romance etc, but random acts seem to have no answers.

Some religious people will say random mortal squalls are the work of the devil or it is Gods punishment for not following his instructions to the letter of their religious dogma. However, a more realistic answer would be...There might not be any logical or rational reasons.

Maybe it just happens to be that particular persons turn in the mortal grinder. If we want to delve deeper, a metaphysical answer can be found for every event under the sun and beyond, but let's not go into that now...Lets keep it simple

How we deal with the adversities will determine how our lives precede in either direction of happiness or sadness. The only true measure of a person's success in life is the moments they spend in a joyful state of mind.

Everything else is secondary trappings such as money and 'must-have' products. Sometimes material goods may seem of primarily importance, but when events go wrong, even people with great wealth will ask... "Why me?"

Perhaps a better way of looking at the squalls in our lives it to say...Thank you for giving me the opportunity to enjoy the beauty in this squall that I am experience at this moment in time... When it passes, I will be far more appreciative for each sun-rise and sun-set that comes my way.

The next time you are near the ocean and a squall hits it, watch the demeanor with which the ocean deals with the discomfort. After the squall passes-by, calm waters are caressed, by the gentle breezes of tender love and exquisite joy.

Don't you deserve to live similarly at ease as the flow of the ocean?

Timeshare

I would think most folks
have heard about timeshare
you can buy one week or
one month fractional share
in a vacation home
mind you will pay a lot more
than buying a holiday home outright
I bet you don't know who
started fractional time share
in the first place?
do you give up?
well it was God
he gave you a fractional share
of time on earth
if you tend to spend time
in doom and gloom
the value drops dramatic-ally
what do you suppose your
timeshare is worth right now?

PART THREE

LIVE WELL

We have discussed eating well & thinking well, so now is the part when we put it all into practice so that we live well.

Become the Hero of Your Life

Are you sitting comfortably, fantastic, now let me ask you a question. What is the connection between a blind lieutenant colonel, a transvestite and a holocaust inmate? It may take you a while to work it out so let me tell you the answer. They are all incredible valiant characters from what I regard as three of the most outstanding movies I have viewed in the last fifty years. More than that, they unify by a potency of powerful strength that you will become familiarized with shortly.

Al Pacino played the role of a character named Frank Slade, who is blind and has made up his mind to have one last fling with a call girl before committing suicide. He hires an impoverished student who is in trouble with his university because he will not snitch on some mischievous wealthy students. As the story unfolds, Frank is in a posh hotel partaking in afternoon tea. He asks a beautiful young woman to dance the tango and the joy of the dance is savored in a mesmerizing manner.

Later in the movie, he comes back from his encounter with a call girl and sits in his limo in dream like divine bliss, savoring the sexual sensuality of a Scent of a Woman (Which is the title of the movie.) Subsequently, the young student stops Frank from committing suicide. He rewarded later by Frank defending the underdog student in front of the whole school with a speech from his heart and soul. It is a delivery of courage and gallantry. It originates from a special place in a human being, which does not stem from academic achievement...A blissful experience!

In the second movie, Cillian Murphy plays the role of an Irish transvestite named Kitten. He embarks on many hazardous adventures and overcomes adversities that would weaken the strongest fighters.

Kitten is a hero who stands out beyond the story line of his sexuality and cross gender. It relates to the true core of his humanity, but the title of the movie, Breakfast on Pluto, relates to someone who lives outside this worlds conditioning. Nothing can take away the strength of Kittens spiritual essence without his permission. He will not sacrifice his true identity, as a joy-filled soul, come what may.

In one amusing and poignant scene, Kitten is posing as a striptease artist in a peep show. A priest speaks to him through a small slit in the booth, reminiscent of a confessional box. He confesses to Kitten that he is his real physical father. It is a lustrous turn of normal circumstances that encompass one of many important messages throughout the movie.

The brilliantly acted story overcomes religious dogma, terrorism, wars, depravity and humanities ignorance. The soul of a human shines through it all and Kittens love for everyone he encounters turns hearts of stone into marshmallows.... A pure delight!

In the third film, we find Roberto Benigni playing the role of Guido Orefice who finds himself incarcerated in a concentration camp with his small son. The Nazi's are going to kill all the children so to protect his son Guido makes up a game of hide and seek. The boy must hide away from the Nazis and the longer he hides the more points he gets. When he gets 10,000 points, he will win a real tank.

Guido makes the words; Life is Beautiful (the title of the movie) take on new profound meaning. If we use our imagination, a little we can see the movie in a slightly different way with the fact that the boy did not exist. We can contemplate the movie from a point of view that the boy was actually his own soul and he hid from the savage barbarism of the holocaust camps by comforting himself inside a place where no harm can befall him.

Even at the end of the movie when a Nazi guard is about to kill him, he marches to his death in a joy-filled manner and winks at his son (his own soul) hiding in a coalbunker. They can take his physical life but they cannot touch or take away his spirit. Life is truly beautiful when the light of the human spirit shines bright...Divine blissfulness!

In all three movies, music plays its part in connecting the audience with the action in a way no words can express. So have you figured out the ingredients that connect all three characters in the movies, and why is it significant in your life?

The main characters all conquered the monsters in their lives by not accepting them as their reality. They lived outside the confines of religious dogma, scientific scrutiny and academic doctrine. You may well say it is only in the movies that people can enact their roles in a fearless manner; however, great directors, writers, actors, musicians and a whole crew of enlightened people who understand the qualities that make a human being human make great movies.

That is why there are very few great movies, for just as in real life, not too many people know how to live an illuminating authentic life free from the manacles of ignorance. Great movies reflect the greatness in humanity. Many people who survived the holocaust have told me they did so because their imagination took the place of their physical reality. Here are a few of the qualities that link them all together.

1/ The pure joy of living can overcome every erroneous action, devastation or hardship that will develop in every mature persons lifetime.

2/ Courage and fortitude are qualities that are inherent in every human being. They are the savory ingredients that add spice and flavor to bland insipid lives and turn the taster into an ambrosial celebrity.

3/ A strong spirit can overcome great challenges, whereas no amount of education or social graces can prepare a person for catastrophes.

4/ Music has profound qualities that can sooth the mind and harmonize with the body.

5/ Love can melt icebergs in 40 below temperatures. Even the most imperfect humans by societies standards can rise above the unbalancing throng of analytical dogma and transcend into higher realities by giving their love to everyone they encounter.

6/ Imagination takes away the obnoxiousness of human behavior and lifts the mind to a higher plateau. A happy face, dreams of faithfulness and incorruptible gratitude originate from humanities image-maker.

7/ Greatness is achieved by good intent to other people. By becoming the hero in other people's lives, you become a hero to yourself.

8/ Ruthfulness, cunning and deceit by others can take away a person's possessions, even their physical lives, but cannot harm the true essence of who they are.

9/ When the mind of a human is illuminated by the spirit of a loving soul no evil force can penetrate the power within.

10/ The majestic grandeur of simple living cannot be bought by the extravagance of money, diamonds, gold or silver. A friendly disposition, a warm smile and enthusiastic childlike laughter are the characteristics and features now playing on a stage inside every human heart.

Mathematics of Life

In a world where, too much,

is not quite enough,

occurrence of unequal equations,

may give cause for concern,

 if we take away six of one,

from, half a dozen of another,

we are left, with zero,

we come in, with naught, and leave… with no-thing,

in the middle,

 the additions, and take-aways,

may lead, to a multiplication,

of abundant complications,
or divisions in narcissistic tenancies,

that split humanity in pieces,

 fractions of friction,

decimals of destruction,

it all adds up,
and in the end,
no-thing is taken for chance,

Living Atop of the Mountain

Ten Secrets of Life.

Babies arrive in this world on the top of their own personal mountain. It is only one-step away; from the paradise, they came from and will return when their innings is over. In this most sacred place, they are in constant contact with their creator/evolver.

Even though their physical body, with feet on the ground, will appear to live on the low lands, amongst the unbalanced assembly of mis-conditioned people, their minds will remain on top of the mountain..

The atmosphere that surrounds their mind is pure and unblemished by any earthly intellectual/egotistical conditioning. This is because they comprehend the mind is not the brain.

It is nourished by a constant stream of universal wisdom that feeds energy into every cell, molecule and atom of their anatomy. A few wise people knowingly live atop of their mountains all their lives despite the fact everyone below is telling them it is impossible to live there all the time.

They are told they must conform by the fallacious plastic conditions of their tribe or society. Fear, greed, anger, jealousy and many other negative emotions are sent their way to try and laden their mind with so much adverse trivialities that it weighs them down and they lose their shelter planted on hallow elevated foundations.

Happily, the wise ones are immune from such erroneous nonsense since a master who drew the blueprints of humanity billions of years ago governs their egos. They say to themselves ...Why listen to unhealthy, ivory tower professors of education, overweight doctors who die of disease, politician with their own agenda, financial gurus whose aim is to line their own pockets or media experts who promote cooperate or terrorist propaganda.

They instinctively know they can tune into multidirectional channels of wisdom projected from eternal sources. With the exception, that they do listen to a few other enlightened people, in influential places in society, who do use their academic knowledge and education as a tool, so that their connection to their architects sagaciousness can be more simply understood.

Unhealthy tasty food is continually thrust in their direction. Enticing dishes are filled with high contents of sugar and trans fats. Because they have kept their brain cells/neurons pure, it will not tolerate such sneaky deceit, and rejects the foods as poisons to their finely orchestrated system. The body replies to the brain with big kisses and hugs thanking it. The body and brain (not to be confused with the universal mind) keeps youthful and fluid as it matures and ripens towards its demise.

Drinks with seductive names are brilliantly marketed to entice weak brains to indulge. However, smart brains favor their minds universal wisdom and overcome the devious ploys. They accept many drinks contain impurities that can destroy some of their brain and body's healthy cells.

So their brain say's no thank you and accepts they may be scorned by the multitudes as cranks. With a smile, they think to themselves ...Viva La Crank!

Detrimental habits such as drugs and tobacco is not an option to consider as a choice, because there is no need of the habitual pollutants to keep happy and contented. Every baby can remain a lighthearted, satisfied moppet of its tailor throughout its life on earth.

It can fashion its existence on tailor-made philosophies that cultivate an abundant, delightful fusion of contentment, peace, joy and love.

They can dedicate their time on earth to help others, whose minds seemingly have slid down the mountain, to ascend the heights once more. In truth, the connection between every mind is never broken and never drifts down the mountain. Its soundness lives on high all through everyone's lifetime. Every mind lives on top of the mountain even though it outwardly seems to have slipped down... It is unjustly muted by the cacophony of ignorance of the ego.

The minds loving, joyful intelligent meanings are overbearingly ignored.

Wise people accept the facts that no matter what mayhem, confusion, turmoil and flimflam surrounds them on the low 'lie-ing,' mortal level, they can live in joy. They understand that they are just one step away from eternal heaven, whilst enjoying a finite heaven within the framework of a lifetime on earths pleasant and gratifying pastures.

Now I had better let you, the reader, into ten little secrets that you may not know and could be why you cannot find any true satisfaction from your existence on earth.

1.   Your mind is not your brain and yet it has a measure of it.

2.   Your minds infinite authentic power can feed your brain.

3.   Your brains limited potency, restricted by its intellectual and egotistical departments, cannot ever feed your mind.

4.   Your mind has no physical presence on earth although it embraces your wholeness.

5.   Your brain does have a physical presence on earth although it constantly sends and receives non-physical communications.

6.   Your brain fabricates artificial intelligence in a range of thoughts projected by its intellect and ego, thus, left to its own devises; it can mislead, forsake and betray you.

7.   Your mind infused with universal intelligence cannot ever deceive, delude or fool you.

8.   Your mind embodies truth and is known by another name/label.

9.   Your mind contains many magnitudes of your soul.

10.   Your soul is part of the creator's spirit.

There you have it in ten simple sentences. An infinite mind, feeding a tiny measure of itself, nourishing a human brain. Now contemplate and meditate on them for as long as it takes to digest them.

You have the answers to every question that you ever need to know to make your life on earth harmonious and carefree.
 All that is now required is that you understand and live what you digest... Where is your mind at the present moment?

Us n Them

In youth,
they avowed
never to get like them,
without ever noticing,
over time,
as dreams faded,
they became them,
and died,
without ever knowing...
the why,
the when,
or
the wherefore
of understanding
to letting go
to let it be
and most of all
life
it is
what
it is

Ten Ways to Triumph over Death and Disease.

It's An ill Wind

The live oak tree became a well-acclimatized, adopted tree in South Florida for many years. It stood up to many hurricanes and torrential storms. That is, until Hurricane Wilma left her devastating mark, making many areas looking like a war zone. Apart from the damage to older buildings, homes and a few newer condominiums, whose windows were supposedly storm proof, the main victims of the storm were the live oak trees.

So what was so different from all the other hurricanes the trees had survived? Well, most strong storms generally come in from the ocean, which gust from an easterly direction. Over the years, the live oak trees roots have grown resilient to strong easterly winds and could hold their ground very comfortably.

Wilma came in from the west with winds constantly gusting at 110 MPH. The trees had no defense in place for this strong attack from the west, as their strengthened roots were grown to resist strong easterly winds. Consequently, they were toppled like nine pins in a bowling ally. Hence, the old saying – It's an ill wind that blows no good.

We will all encounter strong emotional/physical storms and sudden, torrential outside events in our lives, that can wreak havoc with our daily routine, health and sanity.

Over time, we learn how to confront each adversity and it builds our strength of character and fortitude.

As each negative event attacks our serenity and well-being, we dig in our roots firmer and stronger. We become accustomed to each onslaught, and acquire ways of coping with each episode of misfortune.

Many people turn to the medical profession for help in times of emotional distress. They become reliant on prescribed medications that ease the mental stress. Sometimes they receive counseling or psychiatric help. Other people may turn to religion, meditation and spiritual knowledge to aid their plight.

Then all-of-a-sudden an ill wind blows from another unexpected, never experienced before direction and they topple over and die from stress related ailments.

All the past foundations and counseling turned out to be useless against the power of bewildering turmoil and mayhem within the mind and bodies complex systems.

Giving people medication with dangerous side effects only weakens the roots of the body's defense systems and when a more severe ill wind blows, such as cancer, more medication is routinely prescribed. Eventually, there is no resistance from the immune system and the body caves in and dies from a disease. Sustaining life is a valuable and worthwhile accomplishment of the medical profession; however, it is not a cure...

Prevention of disease needs no cure remedies.

Even religion and spiritual intellectual interpretations have no preventive methods to aid people who die from disease. If you study the history books, many wonderful religious folks with high morals and virtues died from a disease.

Likewise, many excellent professors of medicine succumb to debilitating afflictions.

No religion or science could save the innocent victims of any past or present wars. As science advances its technology, it innocently turns the knowledge over haphazardly to those without principled governance. Religious people also misuse their doctrines to annihilate millions of innocent people.

There is no doubting the fact that religious differences are the most fertile source of hatred and conflict. Even so, many people have overcome all the adversities from religious and scientific perversions that have flared-up in their lives. In the holocaust, six million people perished in the concentration camps, but a few did survive. How was this possible?

A wise woman who is now in her eighties told me a story about a time when she was a young girl from Hungary and placed in a concentration camp.

Food was scarce, but when it was available, many of the girls who were from wealthy backgrounds could not eat it because it was not fit to feed a pig. The wise girl told them all they must eat the food even though the smell and taste was repugnant or else they would die. She advised them to forget the past and to imagine the food to be delectable and savory.

Most of them thought her advice nonsensical. Thus, they ignored her counsel and died very quickly. She ate the slop food with relish. Consequently, she survived the dastardly ill wind that uprooted and killed millions.

No style of learning, education, science or religion can prepare any person for outrageous mayhem and catastrophic chaos. They need something else to weather heinous, unexpected attacks. What they require cannot be enacted by a label or pigeonhole from any textbook. Resilience to weather ill winds, which blow from a diverse, aggressive, hostile direction, requires an invisible, intangible power that is storm proof.

No weapon can penetrate its shield. No sword can pierce its protective cover.

It is an inner power that infuses the creation/evolving of the cosmos and since humans are also a strand of cosmic evolution/creation, it makes sense to be guided by its energetic intelligence.

1   Inner power embraces an understanding that it is not dependent on anything the physical, material world can supply. In good times, it's the stuff that breeds champions. In bad times, it's the glue that holds mind and body together. It is a translucent faultless vision that arises in a clear silent mind.

2   Inner wisdom will sift through all of humanities learning and find the few gold nuggets that actually contain truths. This will confirm the accurate path to follow, in the same way the inner awareness already orchestrates in every cell of its being.

3   Inner mastery involves the ability to see through the veil of deceptions contained in all the forms of politics, religion, science, business and other mortal fabrications. No outside influences will cause anger, jealousy or hatred to manifest in the peaceful mind, from other peoples illusionary, destructive schemes.

4   Inner strength encompasses the awareness to disassociate with all forms of human opinions, perceptions, ideas, attitudes, concepts and projects that divide one community from another, no matter how the participants cleverly disguise their plans with a veneer of hope and belief.

5   Inner wisdom understands that if it wears a label to identify itself, that detailed categorization will become the shroud that buries it whilst it has a place on earth and could contribute to the trademark holder's early demise.

6   Inner magnetism embodies an understanding to think beyond normal logic and reasoning. It abides in realms that produce actions of good intent that conform to the well-being of all life on earth.

7   Wherever and whenever possible, the command of authentic thought will intuitively forewarn without fear, when dangers are imminent and will give signals to move out of the way

of impending jeopardy. It brings unwavering balance and tranquil serenity even in the most intense conditions.

8   When it is impossible to flee from physical attacks or abusive mental avalanches, insights into all possible actions will give clear instinctive direction, on the best place to take cover and hide. A strong defenseless stance, that requires no partisan view, will provide safe shelter from invasive forces.

9   When no hiding place is possible in times of chaos, the non-tangible power will give the strength to fight for survival. If physical strength is no avail, it will bring the power of mental fortitude to undertake the task of survival under extreme circumstances.

10   When everything fails to aid the fight for survival, it will no longer resist and will pass away to the home base from which it was born. It will travel from a delicate, eloquent mind, overflowing with love & joy, with a body that is disease free.

Even death cannot take away the power of the true authentic essence within life, which is inside the intelligent energy of every tree, flower, rock, ocean, insect, fish and animal on earth. A person's life on earth is limited.

With each sunrise and sunset, they age and the finite frame cannot hold back the ravages of time. Even the expected demise of the mind and body can be a stressful sad event, for all the people who witness the demise of a loved one.

When humanity can celebrate the passing of loved ones, whilst acknowledging the physical loss, in the same way as they celebrate a birth, they will at last be empowered with the indistinguishable facets that cloak life & death.

No-body, no-thing, no power can remove the multi-dimensional facet essence of who a person is, in real terms, which necessitate no-thing physical, to exist in a state of love & joy. The only one that can dis-empower any person, is the person himself or herself, by the ignorance within parts of sophisticated intellectual knowledge, that has replaced, intelligent, reliable, unfailing energy, emanating from a spring of truthful wisdom.

To live merely with the covers of information that stems from ivory-towered projected academia, will sentence a person to a forsaken existence that lacks true happiness... It stubbornly never allows time to explore the gems below the cover ... It will assign a person to die with all the real treasures still inside them, forlornly unemployed, occasionally misused and seldom appreciated.

The wisdom from mystery schools of ancient civilizations kept their secrets so well hidden, that today, in modern education, the student graduates with glowing degrees, but authentic living wisdom is still a mystery.

If nothing else, every student should leave their place of education with the knowledge that there is nothing outside themselves, which can doom or safeguard them, other than the wisdom contained within their natural, untainted selves. They are and will become their own salvation or ruination.

The aspects and source of people's thoughts and the way the thoughts are played out in daily actions, will make all the difference to whether they succumb to ill-fated gale force ill winds, with broken dreams and depressed minds.

Alternatively, prosper, as masters of their own destiny, with healthy caring hearts and spirited sparkling minds.

True Asset Management

How good are you at managing your assets? Over the past few years, I have received a few invitations to attend seminars at high-class restaurants. Naturally, I have attend a few and enjoyed a nice meal and at the same time listened to expert financial managers teach me how to take care of my assets.

Most of the speakers are overweight and do not seem to be in the best of health. The audiences are mostly elderly retired people and most of them appear to be on medication. Very few seem to be fit and healthy. It appears that many people's wholeness affluence has turned into unwholesome effluence, when it comes to authentic, serene mind and body asset management.

Maybe most people have lost sight of what the real assets are in their lives and thus do not have any ideas on how to manage them. For the majority of people, experts and novices alike, the management of their health, well-being, contentment, serenity, composure, happiness, state-of-mind, body fitness, and genuine love of life is sadly neglected.

Before you tell me that it is the job of the medical profession to manage people's health, do you really want to give up your health and peace of mind in the hope medical counselling, medication and surgery can return what you neglectfully give away? Sure, they can fix-the-unhealthy-up…set broken bones...perform heart operations etc. However, most medical practitioners do not teach their patients how to organize their precious wholeness assets. So who can?

Who can really look after your most precious assets so that you compound your tranquillity and well-being, to earn the rewards of a happy, healthy, wealthy life you deserve? The answer is:

"   Only you have the most vested interest to invest and mange your own well-being.

"   Only you will be the sufferer if you screw-up and get it wrong.

"   Only you will become depressed and lose interest in the things that mean the most to you, when you are preoccupied in all the things that don't really matter.

The only way any person can make sound decisions and satisfactory judgments is by understanding who they are, but firstly and most significantly, who they are not.

Self-examination on a daily basis is essential for any person who wishes to protect their heartfelt assets, whilst obtaining the happy returns their lifestyle requires.

Everyone is different. Everyone has their own wishes and aspirations. Everyone has their own personal slant on life. Everyone should ask the following ten questions to evaluate their asset management requirements.

1.   Do I allow stress to take away my joy?

2.   Do I utilize my time wisely or is it mis-spent on pointless pursuits?

3.   Are my clothes and shoes made of the best natural fibres and do they fit comfortably?

4.   Do I drink enough water each day?

5.   Do I eat the best nutritional food available?

6.   Do I exercise enough each day to keep my body in supple condition?

7.   Is my mattress and bedding the best quality, I can afford. Also, am I getting enough deep sleep each night?

8.   Am I happy every moment of every day in work and play?

9.   Is my mind clear and enlightened enough to make my own financial decisions and do I research every investment before I choose the one with the best value and returns?

10.   Do I recognize who I am, apart from each role I play every day?

Everyone needs to find out if the questions open any skeletons in the corners of their mind that need to be scrutinized. Just like your personal monetary assets, your portfolio of conditioned thoughts requires analysing and investigation.

As with all good asset management, the old thought mechanisms that do no work any more need to be exchanged for newer, better, more interest serving awareness, so the conscious mind can serve you better and produce a higher yielding life of satisfactory bliss.

The more you practice your self-asset management, the more questions you ask, the healthy and happier you become and you know what, your financial assets will also perform better.

If your financial mangers did not perform well and lost you money, you would give them the boot and find better management. So why stick with the thoughts that only bring you depression, misery, ill health and emotions of low self-esteem?

Become your own asset superintendent and manage your resources with gratifying prosperity!

As Worlds Unfold

The words ease into the folds of the heart

be they kind n courteous

or

harsh n angry

is love pressed into the pleats of the mind

or

does hate burn into the skin

who or what governs your domain

your kingdom of peace

queendom of serenity

principality of joy

or

have you abdicated your throne to anguish n worry

your love n joy is always in the wings

expecting its cue to fill your worlds

>   *any moment now.*

Rich In Joy

The word rich has many meanings and money is the least of them Every year Forbes gives a list of the fortune 500 companies that represent the richest companies. They also publish a list of the 100 richest people.

Did you make the list? Well, not to worry if you did not quite make it, for there is a rich list that Forbes does not publish and it is far more significant in the lives of every person on earth... Even people with billions of dollars crave to be on it.

If fact if you asked them I'm sure most of them would give up most of their money if they could buy their way on to the list ...
Alas, money will not get them listed.
What is this authentic rich list? ...

It is a list of people who spend all their moments in a state of joy. Top of the list are the people who spend their time going from moment to moment in higher feelings of blissfulness.

It is an infinite scale to climb and one can never reach the pinnacle in one lifetime. In fact, even if you lived forever (and many religions say you do) you can never achieve peak blissfulness, for it never ceases expanding. It is the live alchemy that transforms a meaningless life, into a joy filled life, for without true joy life becomes meaningless humdrum struggle.

How long will it take you to become a happiness billionaire ...
Well let's do some sums
1 hour = 3600 seconds
1 day = 86400 seconds
1 year = 31,536,000 seconds

I reckon it will take about 31 years and 8 months to get passed the billion seconds of happiness mark ... So you can become a happiness billionaire in less than thirty two years but if any of the seconds are spent outside a state of joy it may take you a little longer.

The good news is it is never too late to start saving up your riches. Even if you only can manage to stay happy for one hour a day that is still 86,000 seconds you have deposited in your memory banks and it will pay you big dividends.

You see the more you save the more interest you accumulate for being happy...It feels good, real good ... Therefore, once you become a wealthy savor of happiness your appreciation for the true treasure of nature will grow and flourish. You may even find your health starts to improve and yes, even your money may start to grow faster.

Set out to be happy for one hour a day and then see if you can extend it. Have contests with your friends and family. See if you can find happiness even in the most miserable circumstances. Remember you only have 32 years to become a billionaire if you are happy 24 hours every day.

If you are only happy for 12 out of 24 hours then it will take you 64 years to become a happiness billionaire... If you are only happy for 6 hours in every 24 hours then it will take you 128 years to become a billionaire... Since time is not on your side can you afford to squander your riches?

Is it time your realized the magical potential of your powerful live alchemy.

So It Goes

It comes in without your permission

The spark of the first atom in the first cell

It leaves without your say so

The final exhale of air

Energies expand n contract

Love's grace smolders on the embers of inspiration

Hate's steam lingers on the icecaps of delusion

What do you do with time between the tick - tock

Who do you sense conducts your orchestrations

Will your life narrative transmit on a high or low frequency

Act's of kindness or drama's of despair

    For sure - it goes before you stage all the answers.

Clear Mind - Healthy Body

Do you view the glass as half-full or half empty. Many self-help experts will ask this question to an audience they are trying to help find positive thoughts. It is deemed if a person is negative minded they will see the glass as half empty.

Positive people will picture it as half full. However, even if we accept the glass is half-full, it may be tainted with toxic fluid.

If we exchange the analogy of fluids in a glass with thoughts in the brain, then our vessel (mind) may seem to be thinking positive thoughts, however unsound conditioning may tarnish them.

We may well believe we are positive minded, but too many times, we still allow negative emotions to overcome our bright persona.

Most psychologists declare it is impossible not to become affective by negative emotions. They state it is perfectly normal to feel stress ... the best people can do is try to manage their tensions and pressures successfully, so that it does not incapacitate them from leading a healthy happy life

To a point they may be correct, however, it is a point that need not exist. If we only view life in a three dimensional, physical world then they are correct.

However, if we look beyond our physical world and contact a more authentic world, that is in the material world but has no attachments to it, then it is possible to eliminate stress and negative thoughts. Are you now wondering how you can make negative thoughts evaporate like snow on a hot stove?

In every human mature brain, there are memories of past events that can spark negative sensations. Over many years, reference points are created and they evolve into a methodical system that perceives and interprets each event that occurs on a daily basis.

Since every person experiences differing events the images projected will be unique to each person. For instance, the thought of a snake or spider may strike fear in one persons mind or a loving pet in another. The person who loves snakes may fear heights while the other person can scale a mountain without any trace of fear. Clearly, there needs to be a cleansing of all perceptions of fear induced thought to be replaced with a more authentic method to process thought, before any real change can take hold.

Let's get back to the half full glass. We can make a quantum change in our perceptions very easily by emptying it 100 percent. We need to empty the mind of all thought ever night just before we go to sleep.

By ridding the brain of all positive and negative thought, we are left with an empty vessel that can gain access to fresh, invigorating, creative thoughts that can bring remarkable results.

True absolute thoughts have no attachments to past events that may hold hidden traps disguised as positives.

We are set free to explore the pure potential of all possibilities. The effect on our wellbeing is overwhelmingly assured. Here are ten points that will help generate the power of positive thinking.

1/ Choose your experiences of life, do not allow them to choose you.
Many events and unforeseen circumstances will come into everyone lives. They can range from the perfect moments to the most horrendous disastrous moments.

Many people's lives are shaped by their experience however, it is far better to allow each experience to pass though our lives like ghosts that walk through doors. As long as we don't hold on to them we can choose to live in a consistent state of delight without any conditions attached.

2/ Love and Joy are your true identity, not your ego.
Every person on earth is constructed from a source of intelligent energy that is filled with love & joy in every molecule and atom. To restrict the true flow of energy with thoughts emanating from egotistical sources diminishes the original life forces.

3/ The first action of the day on awakening is a smile.

4/ The second action of the day is to keep the smile until sleep time.

5/ Understand the difference between illusions and reality. The three-dimension world is finite whereas the infinite world is endless and timeless.

6/ Every day, drink a glass of water each hour (not when eating), deep breath for at least twenty minutes each day and clear the mind before going to bed to get a good nights sound sleep

7/ Wherever and whenever possible listen to relaxing music.

8/ Never allow other people to wind you up, it is always your choice.

9/ Understand education is only a tool for learning and not the source of your intelligence.

10/ The power of positive thinking stems from the power of Joy. Just - Obey - Yourself ...The cosmic infinite self, that embraces the guidance of universal intelligence from a higher power.

Don't abuse your body with greedy eating & stress, rather serve your body with wisdom & truth & it will treat you "well" for a lifetime..

The Cheeky Boy

A guru approached a young boy selling lemonade on a street
corner.
He asked, "How much is the lemonade?"
"Just One Dollar" the boy answered.
"I will have a glass," said the guru and he handed the boy a ten-
dollar bill.
The boy put the ten dollars in his pocket and poured the guru a
drink. "Hey! What about my Change?" the guru inquired
"Change comes from within" the boy replied with a smile

Arcade of Life

In the arcade of life we play with our machines,

an amusement park of desires and dreams

but nothing is in fact as real as it seems,

our world is virtual reality, fed into finite streams.

We are taken for a ride and think we are in control,

when all of a sudden we hit a black hole,

all of our hopes a thief "Time" has stole,

alas all alone, we have to pay the toll.

A pin ball bouncing from pillar to post,

being abused by the devil, mine host,

what a great score, look at all the money we boast,

we are cooking our goose and we are the roast.

The theme park is about to close the time has come,

we've played our last game and have nowhere to run,

we now go back to a place before time begun,

we're about to find out if it has been such fun.

Use this as your Mantra each morning on awakening.

In Love With Life

Spirit's divine love
flows effortlessly though my veins,

my heart beats to the rhythm
of universal graceful harmony,

serenely I walk amongst
swaying palm trees,

with feeling of sacred ease,

heavenly blessings sing in my ear,

my eyes reflect ecstatic universal joy,

cosmic turquoise perfume penetrates my nostrils,

I taste tranquility in the azure sea breezes,

my soul's delicate, luminous touch, permeates my senses,

how wonderful life is, experiencing
the majestic colorful paradise,

on earths temporal playground

Miracles Abound, Miracles Abound, Miracles Abound.

MEDITATIONS FROM SPIRIT

The following poems will heal splintered spirits and refresh broken hearts. Before you start your meditation, find a nice quite spot, sit comfortably and wear loose clothing. Now take a deep breath, now pause, and then exhale strongly. Perform this breathing exercise four times. Slowly read three or four poems with a two-minute gap of silence between each poem. Center on a word, line, or verse and melt into your true being. Relax all the senses and bathe in the cosmic bath of tranquil serenity.

―――――

The Blissful Silence

In the silence of my thought free mind,
I leave the pettiness of condition behind,
I feel the exaltation of God's kiss,
I truly am in a wondrous divine bliss.

In my peaceful harmony I immerse,
Floating weightless, throughout the universe,
I feel the comfort of a glowing ember,
In a timeless world, an ecstasy to remember.

One on one, God as God, in a field of gold,
An endless flowing stream, never feeling old,
Worth more than all the treasure can bestow,
I rise up in an everlasting eternal glow.

In this state of mind, beauty is all I find,
This is the Cosmos gift for all humankind,
It's time to light the sacred torch, don't be frightened,
In Silent Meditation, you will be enlightened.

Early Hours

In my solitude in the early hours
I scale spectacular mountains,
I ascend high noble towers,
I reside in peace-a house of no pains.

In my solitude in the early hours,
For desire I never hunger,
Neither worry nor hate devours,
I feel detached from my torment monger.

In my solitude in the early hours,
Velvet darkness embraces me,
I sense the existence of universal powers,
As I savor divine bliss, empty emotions are set free.

In my solitude in the early hours,
Loves devotion consumes my woes,
Joy descends in illuminating showers,
As I begin to learn a little of what my Spirit knows.

The Land Where Souls Play.

An awakening to dawn mist on the water,
Flowing Spirit's streams to God's alter,
Purifying essence whistles through the trees,
Images of the sacred, blowing in the breeze.

Flights of fancy from birds up high,
Feathers of many colors filtering through the sky,
Sun, moon and stars envelops Earth's dome,
We're all birds of a feather, finding our way home.

Spectacle of mesmerizing movements flashing in the mind,
Melting pots of humans, secrets hard to find,
Love all embracing whispers on the wind,
No physical presence, ecstasy from a light dimmed.

Gifts of joy enmeshed in music and dance,
Visualizing images filtering in a trance,
Warriors in a drumbeat at journeys end,
Back to the womb of creation, active in an essence blend.

Wondrous dreams in the stillness of the dark,
Journey on uplifting voyages in Paradise Park,
Thunder and lightening points the way,
A prelude, to the land where Soul's play.

Treasures of the Universe

Life is an adventure ...with Earth as a playground,
Everywhere we look...treasures can be found,
A ruby in a rose... diamonds glistening in a lake,
Minds filled with beauty...in dreams or awake.

Spiritual beings in human form,
Pearls in eyes...seeing tranquility and calm,
Floating on emerald sea...golden oceans so vast,
Silver vapors in the clouds... platinum breezes as the mast.

Every rock holds beauty in its vein,
Every leaf a different color...no shape the same,
Flowing shrubs bursting...with a glowing love,
God sets the scene...everything is a hand in his glove.

All joined together...one poem in a uni-verse,
Every breath of air...is worth a king's purse,
Jewels of joy...bliss from pole to pole,
Magnificent enchantment...in our universal-soul.

Peaceful Slumber In The For-rest Of The Mind

Listen! How sweet sings the breeze, merrily off trees,
Whispering wonderment, the ear quietly it does please,
Nurturing souls, drifting to Celestial splendor,
Beauty unfolds, as into peaceful slumber, coils surrender.

Castles in the sky, growing columns of inspired aspiration,
Silver shadows flowing through all generations,
Warm cocoons of mortality, linked by silken threads,
Webs of lives, where comfort embeds.

Serenely rests the head of time,
Pillows puff by wisps of the sublime,
Mellow moments spark a fusion sphere,
Perfumed gardens alight, dancing nymphs are near.

Oh, mindful forest flower, rivers many bridges cross,
Branches leaved with neurons, invisible flakes of frost,
Tender is the night, spirits lovingly caress,
Sleep well my children, aware God will bless.

So my friend, there you have it.

Naturally there is a lot of information, truth & wisdom to take in, so be kind to yourself and make the required changes slowly.

You now have a reference book and a wellness guide for the rest of your life.

Keep it in a place where it is easy to access.

Still, understand everything is constantly changing and nothing is written in stone. It is a guide for better choices & the more questions we continually ask, the better results we achieve.

In _Joy!

Margaret & Michael Levy

Your guide to better choices

Better Choices lead to better decisions

Better decisions gives better direction

Better direction gives more energy and power for better actions

Better Actions provide better results

Better results mean a Health Wealth and Wise life.

Everything becomes Better, Better, Better
Who doesn't want to get Better

Who could ask for more?

www.ingramcontent.com/pod-product-compliance
Lightning Source LLC
Chambersburg PA
CBHW071154290526
45787CB00001BA/385